THE DRUGS YOU TAKE

'This book is about patent medicines which the author defines as those we buy over the chemist's or grocer's counter. Drugs and medicines prescribed by doctors are excluded from consideration .... The greater part of the book is devoted to an appraisal of the drugs which go into patent medicines and their merits and demerits are discussed with an objectivity rarely found in books intended for the lay reader ....

'The book can also be read with profit by those who are employed in the health and welfare services and whose work brings them into contact with patients.' – *British Hospital Journal.*

'An unusual publication concerning drugs in that it is written for the benefit of the public and not for the health professions .... It should also afford interesting reading for the pharmacist and other practitioners ... and provides an encyclopaedic index of the medical ingredients contained in the products. In this manner "the man-in-the-street and his wife and family", for whom the book is written, are provided with a quick reference regarding the constituents in the printed formula on the label.' – *American Journal of Pharmaceutical Education.*

'Dr Bradshaw has written a useful book ... it deals not only with the drugs we take but also with the symptoms we endure .... He writes also about the attitude of doctors towards these medicines, about advertising, about the legal position of the manufacturers and of the advertising campaigns which they conduct .... Dr Bradshaw's approach is refreshingly free of professional rigidity. ...' – *The Times Literary Supplement.*

American, German, and Dutch editions in preparation

S. BRADSHAW, M.B., Ch.B.

THE DRUGS YOU TAKE

This edition revised by the author, 1968

PAN BOOKS LTD : LONDON

First published 1966 by Hutchinson & Co. (Publishers) Ltd.

This revised edition published 1968 by Pan Books Ltd.,
33 Tothill Street, London, S.W.1

330 02130 3

Printed and bound in England by
Hazell Watson & Viney Ltd
Aylesbury, Bucks

Acknowledgements

I AM indebted for information to hundreds of people – particularly to those who, whether in the flesh or through the medium of books and papers, have taught me through the years what I know about drugs. I cannot thank them all by name. I should, however, like to express my gratitude to the following persons who helped me with information on particular points during the writing of the book: Mr Gordon Hollis, M P S, Secretary of the Proprietary Association of Great Britain; Mr Archie Graham, Head of Advertising Control, Independent Television Authority; Mr W. K. Fitch, F P S, lately of the Pharmaceutical Society of Great Britain; Dr D. A. Cahal, Medical Assessor to the Committee on Safety of Drugs; and Miss Elizabeth Ackroyd, Director of the Consumer Council. I am grateful also to the Legion Publishing Co., Ltd, for permission to use various figures in Chapter 20 taken from their publication *The Statistical Review of Press and Television Advertising*.

S.B.

To my Wife
who shared all the headaches

Contents

Preface

THIS IS A book about patent medicines and the drugs they contain – that is, the drugs you take, for patent medicines are taken by practically everyone quite often. Prescribed medicines are not considered. They are, in certain ways, very different from patent medicines; and, in any case, their inclusion would have made the book too fat.

It is intended for the man in the street and his wife and family, and I have written it because I felt someone should: there appears to be no up-to-date book for the layman on patent medicines, and yet we spend £70 million a year on such medicines in the United Kingdom. The book deals with the actions of patent medicines, and their drawbacks; their advertising and their manufacture; the attitude of doctors to them; their value to the community; and whether or not their use should be abolished or restricted.

I have used the term 'patent medicine' rather than 'proprietary medicine' or any of the other synonyms because, although very few of the drugs in them are now patented, 'patent medicine' is still the term used by the man in the street for those medicinal products, usually with brand names, that he buys for the home treatment of minor ailments.

All products commonly considered as patent medicines have been dealt with, and some extra kinds of product commonly thought of as medicinal. However, the choice of the extras has to some extent been arbitrary. Thus deodorants are considered, but not cosmetics; tonic wines, but not special invalid foods. A few substances that are not, strictly speaking, medicinal at all have also been considered, such as alcohol and aphrodisiacs. The reasons for their inclusion are given in the body of the book.

Products are never mentioned by their brand names – their 'trade mark' names. It is their drug ingredients that are named and considered in detail. There are two ways for a reader to discover the facts about any particular patent medicine. He will nearly always know what it is to be used for (indigestion, cough, etc.), and if he turns to the chapter dealing with remedies for the complaint in question he will very soon find what he wants to know about his product. It will be very helpful if, when reading this information, he has by him the medicine container or package, so that he may refer to the formula printed on it.

The second method is to look first at the ingredients in the printed formula, and then find from the index at the back of the book which pages contain information on those ingredients.

However, even though it will serve as a work of reference, the book was intended primarily to be read through from start to finish. Only in that way will the reader obtain from it the fullness of any value it may possess.

My qualifications for writing it are that I am a doctor, and that I have spent some fifteen years advising and observing the pharmaceutical industry. However, I have consulted no person, firm, or organization over what should or should not be said in the book; nor have I said anything or refrained from saying anything merely on the ground that the interests or feelings of any person, firm, or organization might be affected.

I hope the book may interest and instruct, and even provide some amusement (where amusement was intended); and that it will prove a lot easier and quicker to read than it was to write.

S. BRADSHAW
Little Missenden

Preface to the 1968 Edition

FOR THIS NEW edition I have brought the book up to date, first, by taking account of the relevant events, particularly medical and pharmaceutical advances, of the last two years; second, by summarizing the provision of the 1968 British medicines legislation; third, by incorporating the changes that time has produced in my own viewpoint. Some of these have been prompted by what has been said by the various reviewers of the book.

To all of them I am grateful, not least to the *Figaro* reviewer who described the book as 'écrit pour un public cultivé', unlike the distinguished English reviewer who thought the style too 'popular'. I have tried to keep both comments in mind during the revision.

June 1968   S. B.

I

The Manufacturers of Patent Medicines

FROM A MAIN road, some thirty miles south of London, a large and expensive car turns down a side road and then, after a little way, into the drive of a factory, one of a number strung along that road. The factory building is large and modern, its great stretches of wall dotted with innumerable windows; floodlit at night, accommodating laboratories and vast offices, as well as some very clean and efficient manufacturing units; and numbering among its various features a staff club, a huge transport section, porters' lodges, lawns, tennis courts, flower beds, and three separate car parks. That large car, however, does not go to any of the parks. It stops at the main entrance to the building, and its driver goes inside. He knows his car will be collected in a couple of minutes, and be taken away for washing and refuelling. He is the managing director of one of the bigger patent medicine firms in this country.

He knows very little about the technicalities of patent medicines, this man; and rarely takes them himself. But he knows about finance and about selling, and about newspapers and Members of Parliament, and exactly how badly the smaller firm down the road is doing since its chairman died last year. He will need all of his knowledge when he goes to buy that firm at a bargain price in a few months. He works in a thickly carpeted and beautifully furnished office, this managing director. He works too, for a lot of his time, in London – in restaurants and committee rooms and Government buildings. He travels abroad about once a month. When at the factory he lunches in an elegant directors' dining room, and round his table he will have, apart from three or four fellow members of the board, a couple of doctors one day (one of them perhaps a very distinguished professor), a couple of directors of advertising agents or public relations firms the next, a prominent M P or a city banker the next. He lives in one of the more expensive dormitory towns near London, and he makes upwards of £10,000 a year. He could, incidentally, make just about as much in any one of half a dozen other spheres, for he is a most able, experienced, and hard-working individual.

This man is, of course, at the top of a pyramid, and there are plenty of very ordinary human stones farther down the pyramid. However, by any standard, they are all well paid, the hundreds and hundreds of work people and executives and scientists in that factory. They work under very modern, bright, stimulating conditions; they are in an expanding company; and the cars they own can be seen in long lines in those three car parks – three because the place where one is allowed to park one's car is graded according to one's status in the company.

This particular firm, as well as patent medicines, makes ethical drugs, for prescription by doctors; it also makes various household chemicals and veterinary medicines; and it has just gone into the business of making chemicals for the garden. Nevertheless, patent medicines supply a good half of its income and the whole structure of the company is built upon them. By and large – though there are one or two important exceptions – its products are reasonably effective, and not expensive, at least if one thinks of that big factory and the three car parks.

But now look at a second firm. It is in the North – in one of the Lancashire cotton towns, like Bury or Blackburn or Bolton, or perhaps across the Yorkshire border in Bradford or Halifax. Its factory is old and small (one-twentieth the size of that first one), and is situated in a dirty back street in one of the oldest slums in the town. One of the remedies it produces is a cough medicine, and by also producing a great deal of smoke (like the other factories in the town), it makes certain of selling a few hundreds of bottles each year.

It is a family business, run by a father and son, with a good deal of unhelpful criticism from various uncles and aunts who have a shareholding in it. One pharmacist is employed there, but no pure scientists; and the thought of a medical man crossing the threshold has never occurred to the directors. The total labour force is thirty-three. There are only four office rooms, no laboratories, no staff club, no car park; and the manufacturing of the six patent medicines produced by this firm takes place in a couple of buildings, each just about the size of a small barn. They're not dirty, those buildings, but the atmosphere is a bit slap-happy.

And the man who runs *this* firm? He also owns most of it, and he comes to work, like his son, in a £1,000 car; but, one way or another, he makes just about as much, does the father, as the managing director of that very big concern near London. His products? They're cheapish, they're quite pleasant to take, two of them are quite useful, and as for the rest – well, if you look sideways at them, they probably do have some slight action in the human body, an action that is neither particularly beneficial nor particularly harmful.

Both these firms exist, but in the descriptions they have been altered in various respects so that nobody may recognize himself and feel unduly hurt or unduly self-satisfied. They are the opposite poles of the British patent medicine industry. And in between there are a dozen other different kinds of firm.

There is the company, a little bigger than the one in the North, situated some fifty miles from London, in a big old house and a higgledly-piggledy collection of huts and outbuildings. It was set up fifteen years ago by a young man with two qualities – ambition, and eight years of experience as a salesman for one of the big companies. It has prospered. It makes ten or a dozen prescription-only items, as well as half a dozen patent medicines; and although about half of them are of some value, they are all much too highly priced.

This firm calls itself X Y Z Laboratories Ltd, but it only has one laboratory and no scientists. Most of its products have been devised by the owner and his wife, with the aid of a couple of books on drugs, some advice from an unsuspecting family doctor, and a very detailed and up-to-the-minute knowledge of what other firms are managing to sell. Some of its products it manufactures itself, but the more difficult ones it leaves to a big manufacturing chemist thirty miles away. The real *métier* of the owner is an Eastern bazaar, where his undoubted intelligence, sharpness, and delight in making a fast penny would find full scope. Off duty – which is not many hours in the twenty-four – he mostly just eats and sleeps; but when he is doing neither he is a kind, vivacious, and well-meaning man.

And then there are the British offices of an American company in the centre of London. The managing director, who hunts, would have liked a certain mansion in the shires as the company offices, but his American chiefs looked at a map and said very softly it was a bit far from London Airport, wasn't it, Joe; and Joe looked at them and agreed. The offices of this firm are really no different from the offices of any other large firm that rents rooms in the same huge West End block. There is a big factory up in Lancashire which not one in ten of the company's office staff has ever seen; and which it runs by computer. It makes prescription-only items, as well as patent medicines, and also – through its subsidiary companies – pet foods, and polishes, and plastic door knobs. Its patent medicines are beautifully made and packed, and they are certainly of some real value. It contributes a good deal of money to charities, chiefly because its American owner is seventy and would like to be numbered with Carnegie and Rockefeller, though he will not be. Its executives are very smart young men indeed, and their rate of dismissal is greater than in any other patent medicine firm in this country.

And, finally, there are two other types of firm, both to be found in the less fashionable part of London. One is a very small firm: it is owned by one elderly lady and two elderly gentlemen, the great-great-grandchildren of the founder; its premises consist of two rooms; it employs five people (a manager, a typist cum telephonist cum despatcher-of-stock cum tea-maker cum receptionist, and three salesmen); it has a single product that in one form or another has been on the market for almost a century and a half; and manufacture of this product is carried out, in a satisfactory, though old-fashioned way, by a manufacturing chemist's in the West Country, who put in the highest tender for it twenty years ago. (The old lady happened to like the West Country, and believed you could never buy anything on the cheap.)

It's a tablet, is this product, manufactured in batches of half a million at a time, and put out in boxes of ten and twenty-five. It is not sold cheaply, and it is completely and utterly useless, although the old lady and the two old gentlemen (and even the manager when he's had a couple of drinks) honestly believe it to be a wonderful, wonderful product. They once asked a very eminent doctor about it, but he was also a fairly polite doctor, and they felt quite all right again in about a week.

The other London firm is a biggish sprawling concern. It has men in its offices who have been making the same entries in the same kind of ledger for the last fifty years; and other men who have been making the same kind of tablet or ointment for as long. Some of its products are useless, though almost worth their price for the sake of the long, old-fashioned leaflets that the packs contain; others are of some slight value; others again are very useful indeed. This company has never discarded a product (or an employee) in half a century.

It has a filing cabinet full of testimonials from kings, marquises, and barrow boys and their wives. It is suspicious of advertising, although it does quite a lot; it thinks tuberculosis is still a major scourge in this country; it has never heard of computers. It has lost money each year for the past five years. It will soon be taken over by a bigger, more modern firm, and will be dismembered: the old men will vanish, the leaflets be laughed at, and the filing cabinet will be tossed out.

And all of this makes up the British patent medicine

industry, each firm having been disguised to prevent recognition, though all the features of the disguises were borrowed from real firms. This book is primarily concerned, of course, with patent medicines, their virtues and their faults; but knowledge of what kinds of firm they come from is not only interesting – it also provides a background that will be useful when we come to consider the advertising of patent medicines, and what the future of patent medicines might be.

But now let us briefly exchange our microscope for a telescope: let us take an panoramic view of the industry. In this country there are about ten or a dozen firms with a very big patent medicine business. Most of these firms also make ethical pharmaceuticals, some of them also make chemicals, some make household cleansers or disinfectants, some polishes, some toilet items, some health drinks, and so on. After these top ten come some thirty or forty companies with a medium-sized business in patent medicines. Most of these companies also make other kinds of product, but a few of them do not. And, finally, there is an unknown number – probably hundreds – of firms making patent medicines in a small way, and most of them do nothing else, at least in the way of manufacture.

Geographically the biggest concentration of these firms is in and around London, though there is also a heavy concentration in the industrial towns of Lancashire and Yorkshire, and a smattering in Scotland, and the West Country, and along the South Coast. About a third of the bigger firms are American owned. The types of premises used are very variable, and the descriptions already given are not in any way exaggerated.

Between this hotch-potch of patent medicine factories and the man and woman in the street who consume their products lie the pharmaceutical wholesale firms and then the retail pharmacist's – the chemist's shop round the corner (though increasingly, of course, the grocer's, the supermarket, and the stationer's are also stocking the more popular patent medicines).

First, then, the drug wholesalers: some of the wholesaling firms are very large companies indeed, one or two of them being connected with manufacturing firms; others are small, family businesses. They deal with prescription-only drugs, as well as with patent medicines; and on the whole they are straight-forward, efficient distributing agencies. They can, however, to some extent influence the availability of products, and the re-tail pharmacists' awareness of them, and indeed they do so. The very popular patent medicines are usually, of course, ordered by the retailer directly from the manufacturer, for the size of his order will make this economically worth while. And this direct ordering is becoming commoner as the large drug firms 'buy up' the smaller ones and so add to the range of products the retailer can order from them.

After the wholesaler – the retail pharmacist, that white-coated figure bending confidentially over his counter or retir-ing to his dispensary at the back of his shop, out of sight, there to carry out some delicate chemical operation, beyond ordinary human ken – or perhaps just to give *himself* an aspirin tablet for a change. The great coloured bottles hang high in his win-dow, cameras gaze at us from one case, we gaze at bottles of wine and spirits in another, or at cosmetics and soap and toothpaste and brushes and combs in a third. But always one will find, as perhaps the most characteristic element in a phar-macist's shop, and usually on the counter and on the shelves behind the counter, a good quota of patent medicines.

Often one can also find on display the chemist's own variety of many kinds of patent medicine – a cough linctus, a headache tablet, a hand lotion, and so on, their containers all bearing his name and address. They are usually made for him by some large manufacturer who specializes in such items, they are nearly always similar in formula to one or other of their nationally advertised equivalents, and they will not be treated in this book separately from patent medicines – which is what they are (advertising aside) for most practical purposes.

What you will not usually find on prominent display, al-though the chemist will provide them if you ask for them, are the 'standard' equivalents of patent medicines – that is, the pain-relieving tablets, the laxatives, the indigestion remedies, the formulae for which are laid down in some official publication, such as the *British Pharmaceutical Codex*. These cost less than patent medicines proper (they are not advertised for one thing), or even than the chemist's own medicines; but they are usually just as good (at least in theory), if sometimes not so pleasantly flavoured or so pleasant smelling. And a chemist will nearly always give advice about them – if, for instance, one asks: 'I'd like something for indigestion, please. Have you any kind of standard tablet?' Standard items are not easy for the lay person to request by name, because their names are often long, technical and unfamiliar, and difficult to pronounce. But your chemist will nearly always help.

Standard medicines (or, rather, the drugs in them) will be mentioned a few times in this book; and, as the ingredients of the great majority of them are also ingredients of patent medicines, they will receive an indirect mention whenever such common ingredients are being considered. Similarly, the ingredients of a few ethical remedies – that is, brand-name medicines advertised only to doctors and pharmacists – will be dealt with: some ethical remedies are known to the general public, are free to be bought by them, and are bought by them quite widely – as well as being prescribed.

As regards sales of patent medicines proper, the retail pharmacist can certainly influence them a great deal. He can display one of them very prominently on his counter or in his window, he can recommend it when asked for advice, and he can even refuse to stock a rival product. He is usually influenced in all this by the discounts and other financial inducements held out to him by the manufacturers; but not always. As well as being a businessman, who sells cosmetics and Easter eggs, and films and hot water bottles, the chemist is a professional man, dealing with powerful and dangerous drugs – a man whose advice on health is sometimes prized above that of a doctor, and who must therefore have a conscience and a set of principles. And it is his conscience that will sometimes forbid him to stock – or at least to display – a patent medicine whose advertising he thinks inaccurate or misleading. On the whole, retail pharmacists are a very useful, conscientious, but mis-understood body of men.

And now we have reached the last link in the chain – the person, man or woman, whom the patent medicine manufac-turer woos, for whom the wholesalers exist, into whose hands the pharmacist places the bottle of pills or tablets: the man in the street. It is for him this book is written – for he nearly always has strong views on patent medicines, or questions about them to which he'd like an answer.

Do all the family, for instance, *need* a regular clean-out? That is probably what one reader will ask. Another will say he sees no need for patent medicines at all; and yet another will say, 'Nationalize the lot,' or he may suggest instead that we could perfectly well get all the household medicines we need through the National Health Service. And to that one can reply, 'Then why do people not do so?' – because the fact is that they don't. Instead of getting them free, the people of this country spend some £70 million a year on buying them over the counter. *Why* do they?

Or, 'It wouldn't be so bad,' some moderately minded man will say, 'if patent medicines could be bought only from a phar-macist.' Or perhaps if the advertising of patent medicines was more strictly controlled, or if advertising of them on television was forbidden, as it has been for cigarettes; or even if certain dubious patent medicine advertisements were banned by law. These are some of the questions and suggestions to which you will find answers in this book; and when you won't find an answer, at least you will find the facts you'll need before you can come up with your own answer.

And then there are those other down-to-earth questions that the idealists and would-be legislators won't ask, but that their families may. For instance: What *should* I take when I have a cold? *Are* vitamins any good for colds? Are they any good for anything, or is it just a lot of nonsense? And what about those pills Uncle Joe is always taking for his liver – do they really give it a jolt, and wake up his liver juices? And then there's Auntie's wind. Oh, and the baby's, for that matter. Ought one to fill him up with gripe water? And what about those travel sickness pills that seem to work wonders for little Sandra – what's in them, and how exactly does it work? And what is in those indigestion tablets Father always keeps in the bathroom cabinet? According to the formula they contain about six separate items. Why not just one? Or eight? Or three?

And then there are the disinfectants that everyone's mother hopefully pours down the drains. Are the hope and the disinfectant misplaced? And those reducing pills the lady next door takes, and that stuff one's grandmother is always rubbing into her rheumatic knee, and the shampoo Cousin Percy uses for his dandruff. Oh, and the ointment his young brother puts on his spots. Are they any good, any of them? And do deodorants work? Or tonics?

These then are some of your questions. And to these, and a lot more, this book will provide the answers – by telling the truth about patent medicines. One very important everyday distinction is between those who have faith in the truth and in people's ability to face it and profit from it, and those who are not concerned at all about ignorance or the mess of deceptions and distortions that life can so easily become. Some individuals, indeed, think life should, quite purposefully, be covered with a cloak of deceit (though they themselves will often wear a mask of honesty and frankness). Some things, these individuals say, are best kept secret from the majority of people. So long as they're happy, why worry? Anyway, what is truth? They believe, these individuals, in 'manipulating' people.

The writer belongs to the first camp. Truth may have to be handled with tact. It is often difficult to find, and sometimes impossible. It is, even more often, difficult to communicate. But one's prime object should always be to discover it, to tell it, to make it absolutely clear – even to the humblest person. Most people want truth, and most of the time they can face up to it, and be better people for it. That is why this book has been written. Patent medicines do not form the most crucial topic in the world today. But they are of some importance to most of us. And this book is an attempt to tell the truth about them.

2

Dandruff, BO, Antiseptics, and Disinfectants

LET US start with the outside of the body – with patent medicine remedies for dandruff and body odour. After all, the outside of the body does come first; and practically every reader must have suffered at one time or another from both these conditions.

Dandruff then. It's a condition in which the outermost dead layers of the skin of the scalp are shed more rapidly than usual, and appear as scales. Of course, the hard outer skin of the whole body is being gradually shed all the time as the deeper skin cells divide and grow up towards the outside. This horny outer skin is shed as small pieces and scales, which in most parts of the body drop off or are washed off. They can't drop off one's head so easily, and they are washed off only once a week or so, when a shampoo is taken. So some degree of scaliness of the scalp is inevitable in the healthiest of people, and whether or not one calls it dandruff is a matter of taste. Strictly speaking, however, it should be called dandruff only when the scaling is enough to be noticed.

A real dandruff is due to a mild inflammation of the skin, which doctors call seborrhoea; and one can have a dry dandruff, or a greasy dandruff – the latter being probably the commoner sort. Nobody knows just what it is due to. One can find various germs on the scalps of people who have dandruff (one can on healthy scalps for that matter), and there is one particular germ, called the bottle bacillus, that doctors used to suspect caused dandruff. This was because in those days doctors thought germs caused practically everything: today practically nobody thinks the bottle bacillus produces anything at all – except more bottle bacilli.

It used to be pointed out, however, that an individual could never hope to be rid of the bottle bacillus because it is everywhere: not just on his head, but on his clothing, on his brush and comb, on his towels, all over the hairdresser's shop, and so on. In other words, if by chance one did succeed in getting rid of every single bottle bacillus on one's person, in no time at all the bottle bacillus would be colonizing one's scalp again.

This, it was said, was why people could never get rid of dandruff altogether. Now, although the explanation was faulty, that last observation is as valid today as it was then; and it is the very first fact people should get into their heads about dandruff, however much they may dislike it. You can control dandruff, you can subdue it, but you'll find it a condition almost impossible to get rid of.

Although it is hard to eradicate, most cases of dandruff can be kept under control by frequent, regular shampooing, and a good, twice-daily brush and comb. 'Frequent' shampooing means about once a week, perhaps twice; though rather less often in women. And this advice applies, of course, to the greasy kind of dandruff. The dry kind can be controlled by less frequent shampooing, and the use of some oil or grease in a hair dressing or a shampoo.

How do regular shampooing and brushing and combing work? They simply remove the scales and probably improve the circulation of the scalp – which is something one reads about in advertisements and is probably a good thing, though one would be hard put to it to explain just why. And using the grease in the case of a dry dandruff helps to prevent the shampoo making the hair and scalp unpleasantly dry (a dry scalp may even become badly inflamed from excessive shampooing). It also helps to 'conceal' the dandruff in between shampoos. A doctor asked the question some time ago in one of the medical journals why it was that dandruff never occurred in countries where coconut oil was used as a dressing on the hair; and the answer was that it did occur, but wasn't so obvious – the oil almost literally damped it down.

Dandruff that can't be controlled by these simple measures should probably be treated by a doctor (though it does *not* lead to baldness). What will he advise? Quite probably a cream for the scalp, containing salicylic acid and sulphur, or salicylic acid and pine tar. Sulphur or salicylic acid helps to dry the scalp and make it peel, and the tar helps to relieve itching. Later on your doctor may advise a lotion instead, containing salicylic acid, perhaps with mercuric chloride or one of a number of antiseptics – to counter any infection that may have developed.

He will also, of course, advise regular shampooing, perhaps with a cetrimide shampoo. Cetrimide is an antiseptic as well as a detergent, though whether antiseptics are of any great value in a shampoo we shall discuss very shortly. It has the disadvantage, has cetrimide, that it does tend to remove a lot of grease and so make the hair very dry. Finally, your doctor may advise special shampoos containing a substance called selenium sulphide. These are often effective in bringing dandruff under control, but they should be used only under medical supervision: one must be careful not to get the shampoo into the eyes, and to remove all of it from under the finger-nails; and if used for a long period, selenium sulphide shampoos can result in the hair falling out and the skin becoming greasy.

But what about patent medicine remedies for dandruff? Well, there are a great number of medicated shampoos recommended – by their makers – for dandruff; and they contain substances like pine tar (or perhaps liquor picis carb., which is made from it), thymol, resorcinol, and hexachlorophene; plus, of course, the detergent that makes the shampoo a shampoo. Hexachlorophene is an antiseptic, and a very good one; thymol too is antiseptic, and helps to relieve itching, like tar. But neither every substance you might find in these shampoos nor every property of all of them will be listed here – and for one very good reason.

The reason is this. A shampoo is always diluted, while

actually on the hair, with quite a lot of water. What's more, it's washed off the head (with pints of water) after a minute or so. Unless, therefore, the medicinal substances in a shampoo are extremely powerful (to withstand being diluted) and either very quick in their action or else the kind of substance that clings to the scalp (to overcome the effect of rinsing) – unless this is what they are, they won't have any worth-while action at all. And in fact, not being the almost miraculous substances just indicated, the medicinal elements in medicated shampoos almost certainly do not have much in the way of a worth-while action on a dandruffy scalp – when the shampoos are used in the ordinary way.

This is not to say that they are not perfectly good substances in themselves. They are. If used in lotions or ointments or creams (as many of them are by doctors), most of them certainly have a useful action; but to expect them to do very much in the minute or two it takes to shampoo one's hair, and when they've been diluted in the shampoo and then perhaps twenty times in the lather, is really asking too much.

But every reader can probably recall someone who got rid of his dandruff in no time by using a medicated shampoo twice a week. The answer, of course, is that he would have got rid of it just as quickly by using a plain shampoo twice a week. As we said earlier, regular, frequent use of a shampoo – almost any shampoo – plus brushing will keep most cases of dandruff under control: the detergent in a shampoo does its job of lifting the grease, scales, and dirt off your scalp quite quickly, and it at least *is* present in a quite high concentration in the shampoo to begin with. Doctors themselves rarely write out prescriptions for medicated shampoos (apart from those of the selenium sulphide sort, which *do* linger on the scalp), but they're always writing them for creams and lotions for the scalp.

Very recent hospital testing of one shampoo for dandruff, which contains a new ingredient (sulphosuccinated undecylenic monoalkyloamide), suggested that it cleared the condition over a three-month period better than a tar shampoo. This is welcome news; but one swallow does not make a summer, and the value of the vast majority of patent medicine dandruff shampoos remains minimal.

And now for a condition even less acceptable socially than dandruff – body odour. Most people believe that body odour means the smell of sweat. In fact, freshly shed sweat has no smell. In other words, if you had a bath, then dressed in a clean vest and trunks, and ran a mile race so that you were literally bathed in perspiration, you would not smell at all. A few hours later, however, you would begin to smell a little; and a day later – unless you'd had a bath – you would smell a lot. And if on the night of the race you took off the vest and pants, having worn them for some hours, you'd find that they too were smelling somewhat.

It is not fresh sweat, but decomposed sweat that smells. And what decomposes sweat is certain germs that live on your skin, and that can also be found on your clothing. In addition, *most* of the smell from a person with body odour probably comes from decomposition, not of sweat, but of shed skin and what is called sebum, the oily material produced by certain skin glands that are quite distinct from the sweat glands. We can call all this material the 'sweat layer'.

But if it isn't sweat that accounts for most of the odour why is it that people who smell a lot also sweat a lot? Because germs flourish best in moist conditions, and so, when there's plenty of sweat about, those skin germs can get to work quickly and in great numbers on the sweat layer. Talcum powder helps to reduce body odour simply because it absorbs moisture: things become much too dry to suit those germs. The only exception to the rule that body odour is due to decomposition of the sweat layer is that in some people sudden strong emotion can very quickly produce an unpleasant odour. How? Nobody knows for certain.

Certain body odours have been thought attractive – though the smell of stale sweat could certainly never be regarded as anything but unpleasant. And from what has been said it is obvious that there are two chief ways of preventing it. One can reduce the amount of one's sweat, or one can reduce the number of germs that will break it down to form unpleasant odours. There is a third way, which cannot be recommended – that of trying to conceal a body odour behind some other smell. This is the way used by ladies who bathe themselves in perfume instead of in a bath. Quite often, alas! the body odour breaks through the perfume or antiseptic barrier; and the social effect can be just about as marked as that due to a plane breaking through the sonic one.

All right, how can one practise that first method of reducing body odour – reducing the *amount* of the sweat layer? First and foremost, one can have a regular bath or shower: daily, if possible, perhaps twice daily for special occasions. This has the advantage that it removes not only the sweat layer but also the germs that will act on it to produce body odour. The kind of soap used doesn't greatly matter. The lather a soap makes is usually more important than any antiseptic it may contain. Such an antiseptic is meant to kill off skin germs, but, just as with a medicated shampoo, the amount of antiseptic in the soap isn't very big to start with, and then it is diluted with the washing water, and finally it's quite quickly rinsed off. For these reasons most antiseptics in soap probably do not make a lot of difference (unless they have a strong, lingering smell, which may mask body odour). However, an exception must be made for soaps that contain hexachlorophene: if these are used *regularly*, the hexachlorophene does reduce the number of germs on the skin.

Don't forget also, when thinking about how you can remove the sweat layer from yourself, that there's also one on your underclothing as soon as you've worn it for a day; so that underclothing should be changed regularly – again once a day if you can manage it, and twice for special occasions. (Alternatively, of course, if you wash it each night and get it dry again for the next morning you can wear the same underclothing indefinitely.) In addition, outer clothing too gets itself a sweat layer – from your body – after a few weeks or months of use, and gets itself some germs; and so will begin to smell in time unless it is cleaned fairly often.

Another way to reduce the amount of sweat on the skin (actual sweat this time) is to apply an antiperspirant substance in a spray or 'roll-on' or stick. Various substances, like formaldehyde, and tannic acid, and salicylic acid, have been used as antiperspirants, but much the commonest and most effective substances to be used are salts of aluminium. They are present in practically all the products for body odour that you can buy over the chemist's counter. How do they act? Probably by producing a slight inflammation of the skin so that the sweat ducts (that is, the tiny tubes carrying sweat from the sweat glands on to the surface of the skin) become narrower, and so let less sweat out. It is now thought possible that they also cause a drop in the amount of sweat manufactured by the glands.

Although there is no doubt that in most parts of the body aluminium salts certainly do reduce sweating, some careful work carried out by an American doctor a few years ago suggested that they do not, in fact, reduce sweating in the armpits. Now the armpits are the biggest offenders in the matter of body odour: they sweat a lot (and produce one especially rich kind of sweat), their hairs retain the sweat layer, and they're hot and moist – in other words, the armpits provide perfect conditions for germs to flourish in. Indeed, some people who use an antiperspirant apply it only to their armpits. And doubtless such people are now saying to themselves that this American doctor was talking through his transatlantic hat, because there's no doubt that, when applied to the armpits, antiperspirants *do* prevent odour. The American doctor, in fact, admitted this: however, he said, it is not because aluminium salts reduce sweating but because they act chemically on the malodorous substances and against those germs that like to live upon the sweat layer. They are acting in the armpits, in other words, as antiseptics, not as antiperspirants.

And that brings us to the second big way of tackling body odour – to destroy or remove the skin germs. Apart from regular bathing and changing of underwear, this is largely a matter

of applying a harmless antiseptic to the skin. (Such an antiseptic is correctly called a deodorant, although the same term is
commonly used for patent medicine products containing antiperspirants or antiseptics or both.) That 'harmless' is important: both antiseptics and antiperspirants must be such that
the skin doesn't in time become sensitive to them, and is not
irritated by them. As with antiperspirants, quite a number of
substances have been used as skin antiseptics to combat body
odour, but hexachlorophene is much the commonest of them.
It is effective, and is found in various patent medicine deodorant products.

By now you should have gathered that most patent medicine
deodorants are of real value, even though they are not the
complete answer to body odour. And now a few miscellaneous
points. As most people are aware, shaving the armpits is a good
way to reduce body odour. We gave a few reasons just now
why the armpits are important: an extra one is that the hairs
in them can apparently 'hold' body odours once these have been
formed, and then release them gradually into the surround-
ing atmosphere. They are a sort of depot for B O, in other
words. However, when shaving the armpit, one should be
gentle and not use strong antiseptics afterwards: it is very
easy to cause an acute inflammation of the skin there.

People sometimes ask whether there isn't a drug they could
take by mouth that would reduce the amount they sweat. The
answer is that there are some such drugs. Belladonna is one of
them. However, they have other effects, mostly undesirable,
besides that of reducing sweating; and in the event, they are
not particularly effective in controlling body odour. Also,
they're prescription-only. For a really bad case of body odour,
when all other kinds of treatment have been tried and have
failed, a doctor may recommend X-ray treatment; but this is a
powerful, and therefore potentially dangerous, treatment, and
so is used only for exceptional cases. Don't run round to your
doctor for a course of X-rays just because your feet smell a
little after a day at the office.

All right, what *can* you do if you have feet that *always* sweat too much? You can wash them every day, change your socks or stockings every day (and wear wool or cotton ones, which absorb sweat), use talc powder, and have two or three pairs of shoes on the go – so that you never wear one pair two days running. Your doctor (or pharmacist) will advise you on what to put in a footbath so that it will 'harden' your feet. And you can wear loose-fitting sandals whenever possible – in the evenings and at weekends. By loose-fitting is meant the sort that leaves at least half of your foot surface exposed and all of it freely ventilated.

However, it must be admitted that there *are* a few people who sweat excessively, whether all over or just in one part of the body, no matter what precautions they take; and who are, therefore, especially liable to develop body odour. Baths, changing of underclothes, deodorants, drugs, loose-fitting clothes – nothing seems to help them. Obviously, when such people are working in a hot climate, they would be well advised, if they can arrange it and can afford it, to move into a colder one. On occasion too a doctor may be able to discover some emotional cause for a tendency to excessive sweating, local or general, and be able to deal with it – or else prescribe a sedative for the patient. And even though it may not be a great consolation, it may be reassuring to such people to know that as they become middle-aged their excessive sweating will most probably cease.

Differences in body odour between white and coloured people, or between different sorts of coloured peoples, is probably due simply to differences in diet. And chlorophyll? We're not quite sure if it has any action at all on body odour. Most probably not.

Why so much detail about body odour? About what doctors advise for it, as well as about the remedies you can buy at a chemist's? Because B O is one of the 'minor' complaints that cause much distress to their victims, and yet it is something many people are ashamed to talk to their doctors about. Quite unnecessarily ashamed, because the great majority of doctors will be only too pleased to help – and they *can* help a great

deal. So, if this chapter hasn't told you all you would like to
know, summon up your courage for just ten minutes, and go
and talk to your family doctor. You'll be surprised how easy it
is.

And now after nasty smells let us close this chapter with a
few words about nice ones – those of antiseptics and disinfectants, the substances that are used to kill germs on (or even in)
the body and outside the body respectively. Many antiseptics
are also used as disinfectants, but a number of disinfectants are
too irritant to be used as antiseptics.

The world is full of germs, and so are we. In water, in soil,
in the atmosphere, on floors, in nooks and crannies; on our skin,
in our noses and throats and bowels, in our mouths, on our
hands, on our clothes – germs are found in all these places. The
moral is that, even though you succeed in destroying all the
germs in a particular area, there are plenty of other germs that
will colonize it again very quickly, so it is often not worth
trying. And, incidentally, life would literally be impossible
without germs, and only a minority of them actually cause
disease: most germs are helpful to man, or are neutral.

Second, germs are living things like ourselves. Anything that
will kill germs will often kill or injure living tissue cells as well.
And the moral to be drawn from this is that one shouldn't go
applying antiseptics to any part of one's person in order to
destroy germs unless one is quite sure the antiseptic won't destroy a little bit of oneself too. Healthy, living tissue cells are
a much better defence against germs than any antiseptic. Neat
carbolic, for instance, will kill off any amount of bacteria in
double-quick time – and any amount of you too.

Next, what an antiseptic will do in a test tube is not always
a sure guide to what it will do if applied to the body; and the
same goes for what a disinfectant will do when poured down
a really dirty old drain – as compared with being poured
into a shining glass dish containing only a few defenceless
bacteria. In other words, 'fifty times stronger than phenol' or
'kills 87 per cent of germs in half a minute' may mean very
little in actual practice. If you must use an antiseptic, at least

use a modern one – like chlorhexidine, benzalkonium, hexachlorophene, and so on.

However, the occasions when the ordinary home (as distinct from a hospital or a doctor's surgery) needs an antiseptic or disinfectant are very few. What is the good, for instance, of putting a disinfectant down a lavatory pan (unless you have a person with an infectious disease using it)? Certainly a disinfectant will in time kill off all or most of the germs lurking there, but on the next occasion on which anyone uses the lavatory millions of fresh germs will be introduced. And anyway, they're almost certainly harmless germs in the first place. What is the good of pouring disinfectants down drains that smell unpleasantly? They almost certainly need cleaning out, and all that is achieved by the few teaspoons of disinfectant that many housewives put in them is a nice smell for a short time plus an unreal sense of security. And, lastly, what one should do for minor cuts and other conditions for which antiseptics are often used in the home – this will be considered in the next chapter.

Listen to what the *British Medical Journal* had to say about the use of disinfectants in hospitals in 1965: 'Anyone who works in a hospital must at times wonder what principles underlie the use of disinfectants. The interested inquirer usually finds not rhyme or reason but ritual and romance. Particular products are often chosen because they were once favoured by a former senior member of the medical or nursing staff, whose memory is thus honoured. It may be that the product smells attractive, or that it is useful for cleaning baths, or that it is cheap. ...'

So what hope for the housewife? Indeed, probably the chief function of antiseptics in the home, and especially of disinfectants, is to make housewives feel more secure and less guilty: using them is like burning a little incense before the god of household cleanliness. On most occasions the best killers of harmful germs are soap-and-water cleanliness, fresh air, sunshine, or a good boil-up. As for pouring disinfectants down a drain – as far as science is concerned, you are simply pouring money down it.

3

Rheumatic Balms and Liniments, Skin Ointments, Acne, Eyes and Ears

LET US LOOK now at certain other patent medicine remedies that are meant to be applied to our exteriors – ointments and creams, balms and liniments, remedies for acne, and various eye and ear preparations. All of these are applied to the skin – the covering membranes of the eye and of the ear drum being essentially skin. However, although that is where they are applied, that is not where some of them are expected to act. In particular, the liniments and balms are nearly always used, not for a skin condition, but for some ailment affecting joints or muscles or ligaments, which often lie a long way beneath the skin.

Some people say quite openly – and most of us feel the same way deep down – that they have great faith in such local applications for sprains, and for rheumaticky disorders, and not much faith in remedies for rheumatism that have to be taken by mouth, such as the various pain relievers we shall discuss in the next two chapters. Obviously, they say, if I have a pain in my wrist, I should rub something into my wrist to relieve it; and if I have a swollen knee, I should gently massage something into the knee that will remove the swelling. What's the good, they ask, of my taking little white tablets? The trouble's not in my stomach or my head.

Now when the trouble is a sprain or a bruise, there's something to be said for this attitude. The treatment should be mostly local – a liniment or a soothing application, some strapping or a firm bandage. However, even for conditions of that kind, due to a purely local injury, you may want to take some aspirin tablets to relieve the pain; and if the condition is bad enough for you to visit your doctor, he will sometimes prescribe a special kind of tablet which, once it's been taken by mouth, may help to remove the fluid in the bruised or sprained area.

And when the condition has a deep 'central' cause (as most rheumaticky conditions have) but shows itself as local joint swellings, local pains, etc., then obviously the most beneficial treatment will nearly always be a 'central' one, even though local treatments may also be of some value. And in actual practice doctors find that tablets taken by mouth – whether they 'cure' or merely relieve symptoms – do the rheumaticky person more good than any amount of balms or liniments. The cause of a swollen, rheumaticky knee, even though we don't yet know exactly what it is, certainly lies deep inside the patient; and the pain of it is registered deep inside him too – in his brain – even though he 'feels' it in his knee. A simple comparison may make the position easier to understand. More often than not, when there's an official strike in the docks, say, at Liverpool or Cardiff, negotiations to settle it will take place, not in either of those cities, but in London. Why? Because the union headquarters are in London, and very probably the strike was decided on there; and because the Government is in London. And that's where the remedy should first be applied – not in the docks, no matter how big the mass meetings there may be.

However, some doctors look down on local remedies for rheumatism because they please the patient while not doing much real good, and because their use is irrational. This attitude is unfortunate. Such remedies do, indeed, make many patients happy; and when the total sales of them in this country, prescription and non-prescription, are probably about £2 million, they obviously should not simply be despised.

Anyway, what is in rheumatic balms, liniments, creams, and embrocations? Most contain one or more of a group of substances known as counter-irritants. Among these are camphor, oil of turpentine (ol. terebinth.), methyl salicylate (oil of wintergreen), ethyl and glycol salicylates, and capsicin and capsicum (substances obtained from pepper). These all irritate the skin, and cause an inflammatory redness in it; and so the patient feels a sensation of local warmth. This is pleasing and impressive, but it doesn't of itself mean that anything is happening in the bone or ligaments where the rheumaticky pain is being felt, for these are often a long way beneath the skin.

However, these balms and liniments do on occasion provide some temporary relief of such pains; so just *how* do they provide it? The answer is that nobody is quite sure. It may be that they cause a redness, not only of the skin, but reflexly in the deeper tissues as well. In other words, the small blood vessels in the knee tissues (or those of the wrist joint, or wherever the pain is being felt) are opened up so that there is a greatly increased flow of blood through them. This *might* result in the rapid removal from the joint area of any substances that have been causing the pain. Alternatively, it may be that, when the person's brain is filled by the sensations coming from his skin (warmth and tingling) and by the smell of the liniment he's applied, there isn't much room left in it for feeling a nagging pain. Certainly the smell of this type of application (that of turpentine or camphor, or of oil of wintergreen) is a very important factor in its success.

Even though we're not certain exactly how these balms and liniments *do* act, we know that the substances in them do not penetrate right down to the affected joint, and provide relief in that way. In fact, it's quite difficult to get substances to penetrate the fatty or muscular tissue and the ligaments round a joint, and so reach the bones of the joint itself.

This old-established idea that the substances in a liniment could penetrate deeply into a joint has perhaps been strengthened by the fact that some of the more modern substances used are salicylates, which, as we shall see in the next chapter, are very good for rheumatism when taken by mouth. However, the kind of salicylates in liniments are not the kind one takes by mouth; and in any case, salicylates taken by mouth relieve rheumatism, not by going to the joints, but by a 'central' action – on the brain.

Another substance that many of these rheumatic balms and creams contain, besides the counter-irritants, is menthol: this produces a sensation of cold and tingling when applied to the skin, and will relieve mild pains, probably by means of an action on the small nerve endings in the skin. Another possible ingredient is a substance called adrenaline. This is a very useful substance when given by injection or inhalation (breathing in), but it probably has no effect at all when merely rubbed on to the skin.

And now a few gentle words of warning. The rheumatic rubs and balms and liniments we have discussed in this chapter are of *some* small value in rheumatism; and the pain-relieving drugs we shall discuss in the next two chapters are of considerable value. However, treatment for a genuine rheumatism should always be started and should usually be supervised by a doctor, who will first want to diagnose the condition exactly. Don't attempt to diagnose rheumatism yourself, or to treat it. Above all, if you're middle-aged or older, and you suddenly start getting a real ache or pain in a limb (as distinct from an occasional twinge), don't assume it's simply rheumatic or a 'neuralgia' and start rubbing in a balm. It may be rheumatic, but it may well be something else: let your doctor decide. And if he thinks you will benefit from a rheumatic balm or cream, he'll probably prescribe one for you. If he doesn't? Well, you'll probably be seeing him regularly, and can ask him about it. At a pinch, so long as he has said you have rheumatism, there'll be no great harm (or good) in your buying and using a patent medicine balm.

The second word of warning against rheumatism remedies concerns those to be taken by mouth and containing salts such as sodium or potassium or magnesium sulphates. These substances are laxatives, as we shall see in Chapter 9, but they are valueless in rheumatism. So are other kinds of laxative, such as the phenolphthalein that some other patent medicine remedies contain. And so are hexamine and piperazine, which are contained in yet other remedies. Much the best rheumatism tablet you can buy (and one of the best that your doctor can prescribe for you) is aspirin. Be suspicious of any anti-rheumatic patent medicine to be taken by mouth that isn't either aspirin or a substance similar to it.

And now for ointments and creams that are to be used for treating skin conditions. First, those ointments and creams that contain an antiseptic (usually with a well-known name) and perhaps just one or two other ingredients: these are quite useful for application to the minor cuts and grazes and isolated septic spots that are common in every household, particularly among children. However, they're being recommended here, not primarily for the sake of the antiseptic in them – because the best germ-killing treatment for small cuts and grazes, apart from letting the blood flow for a time or sucking the wound, is a good wash with soap and water. (And the best immediate treatment for minor burns is to let cold water flow over the burned area for a time.) No, they are being recommended, these antiseptic creams, like antiseptics from a bottle, simply because they do take a little time to apply (and a soothing finger and often a hug are involved in applying them), because they can be *seen* on the skin, and because they come out of a container. All this means that they're much appreciated by children who've suffered some very minor injury or burn, though those first-aid measures we mentioned should be practised first, if at all possible.

Quite separate are the other kinds of patent medicine ointments, those meant for the treatment of skin rashes. We shall come to the acne remedies later, but the other ointments in this group nearly always have an impressive medicinal smell to them, and an interesting colour. This is certainly not always true of the ointments and creams prescribed by doctors; and in this respect it may be that the patent medicine manufacturers are wiser.

However, this is the only real piece of praise one can give to these ointments. It is sometimes difficult to know whether particular ingredients in them, present in small amounts, are included just for the sake of their smell, etc., or hopefully for what they might do to a patient's skin. A single ointment may contain as many as three such doubtful ingredients; and indeed all of the ingredients in these patent medicine ointments will often total as many as six or eight.

Let us look for a moment at how a doctor treats skin conditions, at any rate with ointments. He uses a whole range of them, choosing one for a particular skin trouble in a particular patient at a particular time. He knows that two patients having exactly the same condition may need somewhat different treatments, as may one patient at two different times. Treatment has to be individual.

And then each ointment the doctor uses has a quite strong main kind of action, due to its containing an adequate quantity of the one or two chief ingredients – it stimulates the skin or soothes it or removes the top horny layer or kills a particular sort of germ on the skin, and so on. Often it will have other kinds of effect besides the main one; though if it has, this is because the doctor thinks these other effects (coming from an extra ingredient) are desirable for the particular rash for which he has prescribed that ointment.

Patent medicine ointments, however, even though most of them do possess one main action, sometimes do not possess it to any marked degree because they do not contain enough of the chief ingredient. And the main action (even if one can be sure what that is meant to be) is often befogged by the presence of a variety of secondary ingredients with actions of a different kind, which may suit some patients needing the chief action but will certainly not be suitable for others. (Occasionally two ingredients even have contradictory actions.) Quite often these secondary ingredients also are present in small quantities, and so *their* actions are weak. And finally, the ingredients in these ointments are mostly not very powerful substances anyway, no matter how much of them might be put in; nor are they usually specific to a particular kind of rash.

Now what is the explanation for all this? Well, the patent

medicine manufacturer does not make a complete range of
ointments: indeed, he makes only one or two. But he knows
that, whatever he may say, his ointment will be used for twenty
or thirty completely different kinds of skin disease (not to
speak of the many different kinds of skin it will be applied to).
Also, like the doctor, he is probably aware of how easy it is to
make a skin rash worse. Unlike the doctor, therefore, he dare
not provide an ointment strong enough and specific enough
to be really suitable for most cases of one skin condition (or
perhaps at a pinch two or three): if he did, he'd soon have a
lot of customers, with different conditions, who were not only
not suited by his remedy but were actually made much worse
by it. And as for matching his ointment to individual skins –
that would be unthinkable.

What the manufacturer does, in fact, is to provide an ointment that will rarely do a lot of harm to anyone – or a lot of
good either. He knows that a great many minor skin troubles
clear up anyway in a matter of days, no matter what treatment
one gives them; and so his ointment will often be given the
credit. He uses innocuous ingredients, he keeps the amounts of
them on the low side, and (as he is entitled and indeed bound
to do) he lists all his ingredients on the container (often as
many as six or eight, and including even those that provide no
more than a nice smell) and, as a result, many simple purchasers think his ointment must be a cure-all. Much better
than the doctor's ointment with its mere two or three ingredients. Take a look at that formula – eight ingredients! However, I hope it has been made clear that, because of the nature
of skin conditions and their treatment, it is pretty well impossible for any manufacturer, even with the best will in the
world, to provide satisfactory patent medicine remedies for
them.

What has been said gives the clue to how one *should* deal
with skin conditions. If you have one that lasts more than a
few days, then go to your doctor and let him diagnose and
treat it. If you suddenly notice one spot or patch of redness on
your skin, don't rush straight to a patent medicine ointment (or

to your doctor): quite probably that spot will go by itself in a few days, without any treatment. If it doesn't, *then* go and see your doctor. And naturally, you'll see him straight away if you develop a rash that's widespread, or very angry-looking or irritating, or if you have a temperature with it or any other sign that the rash might be serious. Using a patent medicine ointment will, at best, have little effect or else simply delay you in getting proper treatment. At worst, it could make a mild skin condition more serious.

And now just a few words about what is in these ointments. They contain counter-irritants like salicylates or eucalyptus oil, standard skin remedies like resorcin or salicylic acid or sulphur, antiseptics like chloroxylenol or hexachlorophene, oils like clove or thyme oil, substances to relieve itching like phenol or chlorbutol, and so on. The list is almost endless. But remember, these substances are often present in small amounts; and when there is enough, or almost enough, of them to give something like a worthwhile action, it may not be the kind of action your skin condition needs. Don't run risks with your skin – see your doctor.

This advice holds good, too, for that common and distressing skin disorder of adolescents – acne, for which there are a few special patent medicine ointments. They nearly always contain an antiseptic, such as cetrimide or hexachlorophene, which will certainly help to kill off the skin germs that are an important element in acne; and also resorcinol and sulphur, which help to dry the skin and stimulate peeling. Ointments containing exactly these ingredients, and in much the same amounts, are regularly used by doctors for the treatment of acne, and in this case, because he knows his ointment will nearly always be used for just a single kind of skin ailment (for acne is easily diagnosed), the manufacturer dares to produce a reasonably effective product.

However, there is much more to the medical treatment of acne than the applying of a single ointment. For instance, the face should be washed regularly with a rough cloth and plenty of soap and water; blackheads should be *gently* squeezed out after they've been softened with hot water; the scalp should be regularly shampooed; sugar, sweets, chocolates, cakes, biscuits, and very fatty foods should be cut out of the diet; ultra-violet light, or even X-ray treatment, may be needed; and very often various different kinds of ointment have to be used, and even an antibiotic by mouth. All of this calls for supervision by a doctor; and so the patent medicine acne ointments, though they might well do some good of themselves, ought not to be used unless your doctor advises them. If you have acne, go and see your doctor. And incidentally, as he will confirm, acne is nothing to be ashamed of: it is a common ailment of young people, which can be controlled and, with patience, cured.

And now finally, in this grand circular tour of the outside of the body, let's look at patent medicine products for eye and ear. Eye lotions and drops commonly contain antiseptics – very often boric acid or salts of it, which are such weak antiseptics, many doctors would say, as to be useless. They also usually contain one or more substances (zinc sulphate, witch hazel extract) that will shrink the congested covering membrane of the eye (the conjunctiva, as it's called); and in addition, eye drops sometimes contain a substance to contract the small in-flamed blood vessels (ephedrine, phenylephrine). Finally, eye drops and lotions contain preservatives. However, it is not worth mentioning every one of the dozens of substances present in one or other of these preparations.

It is conceivable that, if one's eyes are smarting and red be-cause one has had too little sleep or too much reading, or be-cause they have been exposed to a lot of dust and fumes, eye preparations of this kind might make them feel a little easier, and might make them look a little less bleary. However, the improvement would not be at all marked, and the right approach would be to ensure that one does get a good night's sleep or does not read to excess or come into contact with a lot of dust. More important, it is not always possible for a lay person to say that redness of the eye is of no great consequence. It *may* be due, for instance, to a conjunctivitis needing medical treat-ment, or to important disease deep in the eye. On the whole,

therefore, it's best not to treat a red eye with home remedies –
eye ointments, as well as drops or lotions – except possibly for
a day or two if you are quite certain that the cause of an eye
inflammation is mild and you intend to remove the cause.

Do remember also, if you have been in an irritating atmosphere, that the eye itself is probably applying the best possible treatment to its surface – a constant flow of tears, which
quickly wash away dust and other irritant material. Above all,
whether or not they are red, if your eyes go on and on giving
you any kind of trouble, or if they trouble you at intervals, do
visit your doctor, especially if you are in the older age groups.
Do *not* attempt simply to bathe away chronic eye symptoms
with a preparation bought at the local pharmacist's.

Ear preparations. Whatever hum-ing and ha-ing there may
be in this chapter over rheumatic balms, or ointments, or even
eye preparations, there will be none at all over the very few
patent medicines there are for ear complaints. Under no circumstances should you ever put any medicine not ordered by a
doctor (or any kind of instrument, for that matter) into your
ear, or anyone else's ear. Drop one word in it instead. The
word is 'Don't'.

4

Aspirin

THE COMMONEST ingredient of patent medicines is aspirin, Aspirin alone very often; but also aspirin with other pain relievers, aspirin with vitamins, with aperients, with antacids, with any one of fifty other drugs; aspirin revealed, aspirin concealed; aspirin with a plain name, aspirin with a fancy name, aspirin with a brand name. Aspirin is, in fact, the most widely used drug in the world, and fortunes have been built upon it in various countries. In this country alone over 4,000 million aspirin tablets are swallowed each year.

Why? Why should aspirin be so very, very popular? Because, as any doctor will tell you, there are two pain-relieving drugs that stand out above all others – morphine for severe pain, and aspirin for mild or moderate pain (which is commoner).) Of those two pain-killing drugs, however, morphine, while powerful, is correspondingly dangerous, whereas aspirin is neither. Indeed, aspirin's properties really make it the greatest miracle drug of them all. No wonder it is popular.

In the case of aspirin doctors and scientists share most of the enthusiasm of the general public. A mere list of all the scientific books and papers that have been written about it occupies a whole book itself. And there is not a month goes by but half a dozen new papers dealing with it appear in the world's medical and scientific journals. Aspirin is of proved value in a great variety of illnesses, and on the whole it is a safe drug, very suitable for the first place in everyman's medicine chest. Never despise aspirin – it is cheap and can be found everywhere only because people realize how good it is.

Aspirin first became available in 1899, though mankind had

been groping towards it for a long time before that. Hippo-crates, the father of medicine, used the bark of the willow tree two and a half thousand years ago for the relief of pain and fever; and willow bark contains substances very like aspirin. The next step, however, was not taken until 1763 when an English clergyman called Stone revived the use of willow bark for treating fever. He used it because, although cheaper than cinchona bark (which contains quinine), it did have the same bitter taste, and so, Mr Stone argued, it might be just as effec-tive in fevers. His reasoning was faulty, but his results were excellent: whatever it was that willow bark contained, it cer-tainly did bring down a patient's temperature.

What *did* willow bark contain? In 1876 a doctor called Maclagan, of Glasgow, found that a substance extracted from the bark, called salicin, relieved rheumatic pains. At about the same time another substance, called salicylic acid, which could be made from willow bark's salicin, was used in cases of fever, the doctors concerned having argued that it would form car-bolic acid inside the body, and this acid would kill the germs responsible for the fever. In fact, it did not behave in that way – perhaps fortunately, as carbolic acid is a poison. It did, however, bring down a fever; and more important, it was soon found to relieve rheumatic pain just as salicin did.

Salicylic acid, however, has one drawback: it upsets the stomach, and for that reason it is not given by mouth at all today. However, it was regularly given by mouth in the last century, and among the stomachs it upset was that of a man called Hoffmann in Germany. Hoffmann's son happened to be a chemist working in a big German drug firm, called Bayer; and he decided to try to alter the molecule of salicylic acid a little so that, while it would still relieve rheumatism, it would not upset his father's stomach. Eventually he produced a sub-stance called *acetyl*salicylic acid that would do exactly what he wanted. One old name for salicylic acid was spirin (because it could be obtained from the spiraea group of shrubs), and a friend of Hoffmann's suggested he should add an 'a' (for acetyl) to get a name for the new substance. A-spirin had arrived – or aspirin, as we now know it; the biggest patent medicine of them all. The year was 1899.

Notice, incidentally, how, between the mid-eighteenth century and the late nineteenth century, interest in sources of new drugs had shifted from botanical plants to chemical laboratories. This change, illustrated by the history of aspirin's discovery, was to prove of immense importance – from it have stemmed most of the major drug discoveries of the last fifty years.

But now exactly what does aspirin do in the human body? Doctors would say it is analgesic, anti-inflammatory, and anti-pyretic, these words being just medical shorthand for saying that it relieves pain, reduces certain swellings, and brings down a high temperature. Let us consider first the relief of pain and of swelling. The two often go together, and indeed doctors and scientists are still not sure which kind of relief is the more important property of aspirin. As regards pain relief, it is tempting to think that aspirin (or a substance made from it in the body) is carried in the blood stream to the brain, and there quietens those parts of it that register pain. It is tempting to think so, and probably this *is* part of the way in which aspirin does relieve pain, but it certainly isn't the only way.

Aspirin, you see, will not relieve *all* kinds of pain. It won't relieve colicky pains from the stomach or bowel, for instance (though it relieves women's period pains sometimes); but it is very good for pains in muscles, bones, and joints, especially rheumaticky pains. And in fact there is always a lot of inflammation and fluid associated with any pain that aspirin relieves. The big joint swellings that occur in rheumatic fever, for instance, vanish remarkably quickly once the patient is given aspirin. In other words, a part of aspirin's pain-relieving effect is probably due to its anti-inflammatory action in causing a reduction of swelling and tension at the point where the pain is felt – even though we do not know exactly *where* it acts to produce this effect.

As regards most minor aches and pains, if they are not relieved by one or two tablets of aspirin there'll be no good giving the patient another couple of tablets in the hope that the bigger dose will do the trick – it won't. This does not mean there aren't some patients who will be told by their doctors to take a bigger dose (they will need it for aspirin's anti-inflammatory, not its pain-relieving, action); or that a dose every four hours or so may not sometimes be needed.

Incidentally, it isn't easy to prove conclusively that aspirin (or other analgesic drug) really does relieve pain, at least by truly scientific tests in a laboratory. And a difficulty in clinical testing is that, if you give a plain sugar tablet to a hundred people complaining of a minor pain, but without telling them what the tablet is, thirty or forty of them will say the tablet *has* relieved their pain. And it has – or at any rate the pain has gone. Time may be a great healer, but faith is an even greater one. However, in the case of aspirin the fact that millions of people over a period of many years have said it certainly does relieve their pain – this is the best possible proof that it does have a genuine pain-relieving action.

Aspirin's third property is its power to reduce a high temperature. The best way to bring down a fever, of course, is to find the cause, if one can, and then deal with it, if possible; and germs are the usual cause of a fever – as in pneumonia, or typhoid fever, or meningitis. The germs of such serious diseases can usually be destroyed or subdued with drugs like penicillin or the sulpha drugs; but there are a number of less dangerous 'fevers' (the common cold, for instance, or influenza, or many sore throats) in which the germs are either not affected by such drugs, or else are not dangerous enough to justify their use – because, after all, such drugs can be expensive, and can sometimes be dangerous themselves. These less serious fevers are those that we commonly treat at home ourselves with a patent medicine, and it is for them that aspirin is often used.

How does aspirin bring down a raised temperature? Probably by causing extra water to enter the blood stream, this in turn leading to increased sweating and to an opening up of the small blood vessels in the skin. These, of course, are the effects produced by vigorous exercise, and they result in the body losing extra heat, and so – in the case of a fever – its temperature comes down. Whether bringing down the temperature in such minor conditions as the common cold does any good (apart from making the patient *feel* easier for a time) nobody knows. Conceivably it could do harm, for a raised temperature is, after all, one of the means the body uses to help kill off the germs that have invaded it.

However, using aspirin to bring down the temperature in minor ailments cannot be doing any *great* harm; and people will certainly go on using it, no matter what any doctor may say. Incidentally, what people with a fever mostly want when they take aspirin is relief from the aches and pains that almost inevitably go with fevers; but as well as providing relief from aches and pains, aspirin will bring down the temperature. One cannot separate the two actions.

Although aspirin will reduce a high temperature, it has no effect on a normal one. In other words, there is no point in taking it on a hot summer's day in the hope that it will make you feel any cooler – it won't. Another important thing to remember about the action of aspirin is that it doesn't quieten one's nerves at all, or help one to go to sleep the way barbiturate drugs do; and it doesn't make one feel unreasonably cheerful, as some other drugs do – morphine, for instance. It is because they possess one or both of these actions that certain drugs are drugs of addiction; and it is because aspirin does not possess them that people never get addicted to it. And finally in this catalogue of virtues, aspirin has no bad effect on the heart. In fact, although this is claimed as a special virtue for some aspirin products, nobody now believes that aspirin *does* have such an effect; and so to say it hasn't is rather like a car manufacturer claiming that his new model will never turn round and bite you.

So far we have done little but praise aspirin. Has it no drawbacks then, this remarkable drug? Yes, it has. Every drug that has ever existed has drawbacks. A few people are allergic (or hypersensitive) to aspirin. When they take a tablet – or even if they put a few grains of aspirin on the tongue – they come out

in a nettle rash, or else develop an attack of asthma. Such
people soon learn to avoid taking aspirins as such. Unfortunately they can't always be sure that some medicine they're
thinking of taking does not contain aspirin. Two doctors in a
London teaching hospital recently compiled a list of most products available in this country or the U S A containing aspirin,
or salicylates, in one form or another. (Salicylates are salts of
salicylic acid, and are rather like aspirin.) Well, how many do
you think there were? The answer is almost four hundred.
This is both a tribute to the value of aspirin, and a warning to
anyone who is allergic to it to make absolutely sure before
taking a strange patent medicine that there is no aspirin or
other salicylate in it. If in doubt, you should ask a doctor or a
pharmacist.

Aspirin's second defect is that some people suffer from
nausea, vomiting and stomach discomfort after taking it. With
some of them this upset is purely psychological. They will say,
for instance, that one special make of aspirin does not upset
their stomachs, but certain other makes do. Now, as far as
doctors are concerned, there is usually no difference at all between the aspirin that doesn't cause upset in these people and
those that do – apart from the name on the label and the price.
And indeed, if they are given a tablet of one of the 'upsetting'
aspirins, but believe it is the 'safe' kind, they will often suffer
no stomach upset at all.

However, not all stomach upset caused by aspirin is of this
psychological kind. Some of it is a genuine effect of aspirin
itself, perhaps due to irritation of the stomach lining by aspirin.
'Perhaps' is the right word because, although aspirin certainly
can irritate the stomach, the stomach symptoms it causes may
arise after the aspirin has been absorbed from the stomach
and intestines into the body. The aspirin, having been carried
to the brain in the blood stream, may be stimulating a part of
the brain concerned with vomiting – and so the person vomits.

This may seem to be a very far-fetched explanation, but it
does explain one small fact that will not fit with the 'stomach
irritation' theory; if one injects a salicylate (and aspirin is

really a salicylate of a special kind) into a person's vein, vomiting can be very quickly produced. Now clearly this vomiting could not be due to irritation of the stomach lining, because the salicylate has not been put into the stomach. It has been put into a vein, from which it will very quickly reach the brain; and presumably it has caused the vomiting by an action on the brain. Similarly ointments containing salicylic acid occasionally cause nausea, due to the acid being absorbed through the skin and carried to the brain. All this may seem bizarre, but then a new idea often does.

Anyway, much the most important undesirable effect of aspirin is that it causes, not just stomach irritation, but bleeding from the stomach or intestines. Indeed, we know that 70 per cent of normal people have some bleeding when taking an aspirin preparation in fairly big doses. This too may be difficult to credit, but it has been proved beyond all doubt. You wouldn't notice the bleeding because the usual amount of blood lost is only about a teaspoonful a day on average, and by the time it passes out of the body – which will be the next time the bowels are opened – it is not bright red but has become dark in colour, and has been mixed up with the motion. In fact, because it isn't easy to detect, such blood is known to doctors as occult (or hidden) blood.

Certain special chemical tests, however, can show up small amounts of blood in the motions, and as long ago as 1916 they showed that people receiving salicylates were often losing blood. This was obviously important, or so it seems to us today; and yet nothing further was done until 1938 when two doctors at Guy's Hospital, London, examined the stomachs of a number of people after they had taken an aspirin tablet. They did this very simply with a special, slim, illuminated tube, called a gastroscope, which is passed down the patient's gullet. When these doctors passed this instrument into the stomachs of people who had just taken aspirin, they saw that in most cases the lining was obviously inflamed, and in some there was actual bleeding. So it was pretty clear where the blood found in the stools was coming from.

It may sound incredible, but yet again little further work was carried out on this subject until the 1950s – although in the last fifteen years dozens of scientific papers dealing with it have been published. And what have they proved, these new papers? First, that *every* known variety of aspirin causes bleeding from the stomach or intestine. Two kinds, a fizzy aspirin and an aluminium aspirin, cause less bleeding than the others; but no aspirin is free from this fault. (Giving aspirin a special coating also reduces the bleeding, but then the aspirin may not be properly absorbed.) Second, curiously enough, there seems to be little connection between the indigestion caused by aspirin and the bleeding caused by it. In other words, a person may be losing only a little blood each time he takes an aspirin tablet, but may have a lot of indigestion from aspirin; or he may have been having no indigestion at all from it, and yet one day will lose a lot of blood.

Third, aspirin does occasionally cause a really big bleed: the patient may vomit blood or pass a lot of altered blood in his motions. This, we now know, can happen in people with no previous symptoms of indigestion and no signs of a peptic ulcer. Indeed, in the great majority of healthy people who have a big bleed aspirin is the cause. And it can occur after a single dose as well as in someone taking aspirin over a period. Patients with a peptic ulcer seem to be only a little more liable to one of these big bleeds after taking aspirin; but in about one third of *all* big bleeds (that is, in ulcer and non-ulcer patients) aspirin is to blame. Liability to a big bleed is not tied up with any special tendency to the small bleeds already mentioned.

One difficulty in investigating this matter has been that so many people take aspirin so very often that, unless one is careful, it would be possible to think aspirin had all kinds of effect that, in fact, have nothing at all to do with it. For instance, perhaps half the people who have won a big prize on the football pools have taken an aspirin tablet in the fortnight before they won it. Did the aspirin make them win? No, obviously not, because half the people who didn't win would be found to have taken aspirin also. In that instance very few of us would think aspirin had had any effect; but there are other instances where the cleverest of scientists can go wrong. However, despite difficulties of this kind, there is now no doubt at all that *every* kind of aspirin causes bleeding. (And incidentally, aspirin prescribed by a doctor – and it is prescribed very often – is exactly the same as aspirin in patent medicine form.)

What is it that causes the stomach to bleed after aspirin? Probably it is irritation of the stomach lining. Aspirin causes the cells of this lining to be shed a lot more quickly than usual, which would make small ulcers of the lining more likely. Such ulcers, which may heal very quickly, have been seen in some patients with a big bleed but no previous indigestion, and also in those who have just a slight ooze when taking biggish doses of aspirin over a period. Nobody yet knows why only 70 per cent of people have such an ooze, and why very occasionally a healthy person should have a big bleed after aspirin. Probably in the latter sort of person the stomach lining has become very sensitive to aspirin for a short time.

It used to be thought that it was solid particles of aspirin that did the damage: a doctor who passed a gastroscope tube in a patient who had just taken an aspirin tablet would often see in the stomach small areas of inflammation round little pieces of the tablet. Sometimes there would even be a small ulcer of the stomach corresponding in shape to a piece of tablet. It was because of findings like this that doctors believed for some time that soluble aspirin did not cause any bleeding. However, since we now know that bleeding is caused by *all* kinds of aspirin – including soluble aspirin – any irritation of the stomach lining can apparently be caused by a solution of aspirin as well as by a tablet, though perhaps a tablet is rather more severe in its effect.

And what is the practical importance of this effect of aspirin? First, occasional use of aspirin is perfectly safe for most of us. However, the small loss of blood caused by biggish doses may well, over a long period, produce anaemia, especially in women. So never go on taking daily aspirin for more than a few days except on a doctor's orders. (Of course, another excellent reason for not doing so is that any condition serious enough to make you *want* to take a drug for day after day should always be diagnosed and treated by a medical man.) Second, people who suffer from a peptic ulcer or from indigestion due to some other cause should not take aspirin tablets at all unless advised to do so by their doctor. Thirdly, do always take aspirin crushed up in some liquid, and preferably with a meal; and if not with a meal, then with a good drink of water or milk. Fourth, do not take aspirin if your stomach is upset in any way, and particularly not if this upset is due to alcohol.

We have spent a lot of time on this topic of bleeding and indigestion caused by aspirin because it is a very interesting story. But we must not get it out of perspective. Enormous quantities of aspirin, prescribed and in patent medicine form, are taken every year, and yet one is not hearing all the time of people being made seriously ill by it. Provided one abides by the four simple rules that have just been mentioned, there is certainly no great harm in taking aspirin now and again, and there can be a great deal of good in it. Tens of thousands of headaches and minor aches and pains are relieved by aspirin every day; and it is a standard form of medical treatment for practically all kinds of rheumatism. Indeed, on the average it is probably as valuable in rheumatoid arthritis as cortisone and similar powerful drugs, which have much more serious drawbacks. So don't throw your aspirins away, but equally don't eat them like sweets.

One good reason for not doing so is that there are some 12,000 cases of poisoning each year in England and Wales due to aspirin overdosage. In view of the total national consumption of aspirin, this is not a disproportionate number: it would be expected from any fairly powerful drug that was to be found in most households. Nevertheless, and although there is an effective method of treating aspirin poisoning, it does kill over 200 people a year in England and Wales, some of them children; and we should keep aspirin – like all other medicines –

out of reach of little children, and never give aspirin to a young child except on a doctor's advice.

Are plain, standard aspirin tablets as good as branded aspirin tablets? It depends on who makes the standard aspirin tablets; and, of course, one can't always tell who did. The aspirin itself is the same; but as with most standard tablets, the aspirin kind is sometimes inferior in all sorts of minor ways to branded aspirins, and sometimes it is just as good. Inferior because of impurities or decomposition or the way the tablet has been made, and so on: the manufacturer of a branded tablet wouldn't dare risk his good name by putting out such tablets. For some people these minor defects in some standard aspirin tablets can add up to a quite considerable drawback, so that they often think it worth paying the considerably higher price charged for the branded than for the standard item.

It has been said of morphine and aspirin that man made aspirin but morphine came from heaven. However, it would be a courageous person who would venture to say which of the two has been of the greater value to mankind. Yet morphine, or the opium from which it is made, has been available for centuries, whereas aspirin is younger than many people alive today. And if aspirin hasn't saved the lives of many of them, it has at one time or another made life easier for practically every single one of us.

5

Other Pain Relievers

THOUGH SOME patent medicine analgesics contain nothing but aspirin (plain, or else in soluble or buffered form), a lot of them contain other drugs as well, these other drugs being often, but not always, mild pain relievers. And a few patent medicine analgesics contain no aspirin at all, but one or more of these other pain-relieving drugs instead.

The reason usually given for these mixtures of two or three drugs is that only small amounts of the drugs are present and these are much less likely to cause undesirable 'side effects' than the large amount of any one drug needed to give the same pain-relieving effect. This is probably true, but the real reason, one suspects, for such mixtures, is that the majority of mankind still believe that the more ingredients there are in any one medicine the better it must be. It's chiefly doctors who think more highly of a medicine if it contains just one substance; and only during the last twenty years or so that even they have begun to think in this way.

However, analgesic *pot-pourris* aren't going to vanish because some doctors disapprove of them; and the commonest of those other pain-relieving drugs in them is phenacetin, sometimes called acetophenetidin – just as you will sometimes find aspirin itself described on a label as acetylsalicylic acid, which is its less familiar, chemical name. Phenacetin is derived from acetanilide, the value of which was discovered in one of those absurd, chance ways that can so often be found in the history of medicine. A patient who had worms was given it in mistake for another drug. And acetanilide cured the worms? Not at all. It didn't affect the worms, but this patient happened, quite by chance, to have a fever as well, and acetanilide brought the fever down remarkably. Phenacetin was developed from acetanilide a little later.

As well as bringing down a high temperature, phenacetin, like aspirin, relieves pain and reduces inflammation. However, unlike aspirin, it also causes very slight relaxation and drowsiness – in other words, it is a very mild sedative – and that is why it has proved a good drug for the relief of headaches, which are often caused by a person being 'tensed up'. Phenacetin is not as good as aspirin for rheumatic complaints.

And drawbacks? If used over a long period, phenacetin can cause an undesirable change in the colouring of the blood, so that people taking it look greyish blue. It can also cause an anaemia, and even a headache – for which, of course, the person concerned then takes more phenacetin. ... Even more important, prolonged consumption of phenacetin can have a serious harmful effect on the kidneys. It is for these reasons that many doctors, including the writer, think we could probably do without phenacetin altogether. (There is, incidentally, some interesting recent evidence that the kidney may be harmed, not only by phenacetin, but by biggish doses of aspirin or caffeine.)

In some patent medicines phenacetin is combined with aspirin and with codeine, just as it is in the Codeine Co. tablets that many people buy, thinking them stronger and better than plain aspirin because of the codeine they contain. It isn't surprising that they're stronger as they contain almost as much aspirin as an ordinary aspirin tablet *plus* the same amount of phenacetin. But they contain very little codeine: in fact, it has been said that the amount of codeine in them is sufficient to cause constipation, though not enough to relieve pain.

What is this substance, codeine? In the right doses it is a moderately strong pain-relieving drug, derived from opium, as morphine is. However, unlike morphine, it has practically no psychological effects – it doesn't make one unduly cheerful. And as it is mostly effects of this kind that make morphine (and other substances) into drugs to which one can become an addict, people are very much less likely to become addicted to codeine. Nevertheless, there are certain restrictions on the sale of codeine, at least in largish quantities; which is why the compound analgesics we've been discussing do not contain much of it. Incidentally, this codeine in pain-relieving tablets is the same codeine as occurs in the Linctus Codeine used for coughs.

One relatively new analgesic that is coming to be used more and more in patent medicines is called paracetamol. It has been known for many years, but it is only during the last ten years or so that – thanks to the enterprise of one pharmaceutical company – it has been at all widely used. When phenacetin is absorbed into the body, it breaks down chemically to paracetamol, and it is the paracetamol that gives phenacetin its pain-relieving properties. However, unlike phenacetin, paracetamol does not have any undesirable effects on the kidneys or the blood. Much more important (at least from the viewpoint of some patent medicine manufacturers), it does not cause indigestion or stomach bleeding as aspirin does. Indeed, the great success of paracetamol in recent years has not been due to any positive virtues it has, but to its apparent lack of vices. Every time there was a mention in a newspaper of what aspirin did to the stomach, a number of readers would go and ask their chemists what they could take instead – and 'paracetamol' was the usual answer.

How good an answer was it, in fact? Well, paracetamol is almost as effective in relieving pain as aspirin, but it is not nearly as good at reducing inflammation, so that paracetamol is not the right drug for treating most cases of rheumatism – unless, of course, the patients are being badly upset by aspirin. And then paracetamol does have *some* faults. It occasionally has a serious toxic effect on the blood, and overdosage is certainly harmful. Moreover, we do not know nearly as much about the nature of paracetamol poisoning and its treatment as we do about aspirin poisoning. This point was made in the correspondence columns of the *British Medical Journal* following a suggestion that, because of aspirin's undesirable effects on the stomach, paracetamol should replace it as a reliever of everyday aches and pains in the ordinary household. The time for any such change is not yet.

There are two other drugs that are similar to aspirin and that are sometimes used in patent medicine analgesics. One is sodium salicylate, a much older drug than aspirin. It is still very often prescribed by doctors for the treatment of rheumatic fever, but it is not as good as aspirin at relieving ordinary aches and pains, and it certainly upsets the stomach. The other is called salicylamide, and, as well as being a mild analgesic like aspirin, it will also quieten people's nerves a little, just as phenacetin will. Indeed, the two of them have been used together as a mild patent medicine sedative. Salicylamide, however, has the drawback that the body gets rid of it very quickly indeed, so that it is almost impossible to get a high level of it in the blood.

Another drug, but of a quite different kind, that is often combined with aspirin and phenacetin is caffeine. Caffeine is not primarily a pain-relieving drug at all, although it does appear to relieve tension headaches on occasion. As most people know, it is the substance in tea and coffee that provides the slight 'lift' people get from these beverages; and it is combined with aspirin and phenacetin because these two drugs – phenacetin particularly – have a slight depressing effect on the nervous system. This does not mean they make people feel depressed or down in the dumps. It means that the substances concerned 'quieten' the nerve tissues a little; and it is because of this action that phenacetin makes people feel a shade more relaxed, or even slightly sleepy. Obviously this would be undesirable for people who have to carry on with a day's work, and so caffeine with its kick is included to counteract this tendency. However, the amount included is often very small, and, in any case, the depressing effect of ordinary doses of analgesics is unimportant. We shall take a closer look at caffeine in Chapter 16.

Finally, quinine is a common component of patent medicine analgesics, especially if they are meant to be used chiefly for patients with mild fevers, like colds and 'flu. Quinine's greatest value, of course, is in the treatment of malaria; but it also acts as a bitter (see Chapter 7), and it will help to bring down a high temperature, no matter what the cause. It is doubtful, however, if the small amounts of quinine present in certain patent medicines really add much to the effect of drugs like aspirin or phenacetin. Indeed, the provision of quinine for patients with a fever is largely a matter of tradition; and as it is a substitute that can occasionally cause serious reactions, it would probably be best for quinine to be dropped from most patent medicines.

Its use over the centuries does, however, illustrate nicely the way the wheel of medical fortune turns. You may remember the eighteenth-century clergyman who gave willow bark to a patient with a fever because it had the same bitter taste as the highly prized cinchona bark (the source of quinine) but was cheaper than it. Nowadays quinine is much cheaper than cinchona bark was, and so the patent medicine manufacturers are able to add it with hardly a thought to our modern miracle drug, aspirin – the enormously successful descendant of that humble eighteenth-century willow bark.

And now, before we leave this business of analgesic drugs, some commonsense advice about pain and how to deal with it. First and foremost, you should go to your doctor if ever you have an unusual pain that has not got some minor obvious cause, or if your pain lasts a long time, or if you're in any real doubt as to whether it's the kind of pain you can treat yourself. It is a truism to say that pain is nature's warning signal, but then statements become truisms only if they express a truth so important to man that it must be repeated over and over again. Pain *is* a warning signal, though there are others; and it should not be ignored. Not all pain means that one has some serious illness: the majority of pains respond quite quickly to quite simple measures. But, if you are in any doubt, do let your doctor decide what the cause is, and what the treatment should be.

On the other hand, we all get plenty of *little* aches and pains, particularly when we become middle-aged, which can be treated with homely remedies – provided a doctor has assured us, when we first experienced the particular kind of pain, that it was due, say, to a mild muscular rheumatism, or, in the case of a headache, that it was due to worry. Once you get to know these little pains you shouldn't need to bother the doctor with them every time they afflict you.

However, what you should do is to try to imitate what a doctor always does when faced by a patient complaining of pain (or of any other symptom, for that matter). He tries to find out what the cause is. Don't rush straight to your favourite analgesic tablet. Stop for a few moments and think what has probably brought on your pain. If it's a headache you have, ask yourself whether you've been particularly worried or upset or overworked – because a headache is easily brought on if one gets 'tensed up', and then the correct treatment is not merely to take a pain-relieving tablet but also to try and rid oneself of whatever had caused the tension, and to avoid it in future.

If it's a pain in the muscles or joints that you've got, ask yourself if it wasn't brought on by that sudden spring spurt of gardening the day before, or by that extra set of tennis. If so, then as well as an aspirin or two, you'll be well advised to take only a small amount of exercise for a couple of days, or perhaps even to rest. However, although rest is a good treatment for many kinds of pain, it is not *always* required. The chronic aches of an arthritis, for instance, are best kept at bay by regular small amounts of exercise, no matter how stiff one's joints may feel when one first steps out. If one doesn't exercise the stiff joints, they may 'seize up'.

Another quite good method of treatment for most kinds of pain is to apply heat to the painful part, either by wrapping it up well, or by means of a hot water bottle, or – in the case of rheumaticky pains – by applying a liniment or balm. And when applying a balm – use a little massage as well, for this too is an excellent way of tackling muscle and joint pains.

However, even if you have found the cause of your pain and have treated it accordingly, and have used rest and heat and massage, you will probably still want to take an analgesic; so here are a few tips. The first one is chiefly for parents (though many mothers and fathers will have worked it out for themselves already). There are two parts to any pain: the pain itself, and the person's reaction to it. Often this reaction – the tension and anxiety and the surprise associated with the pain – are more important than the pain itself, and this is particularly true in children. Correspondingly, although a good analgesic tablet *will* relieve pain, it will not always relieve these associated and often more important accompaniments of pain.

They will go in no time, of course, once the pain has gone; but they can often be quite quickly relieved if the person providing the tablet (the doctor or nurse, or the parent when it is a child who is suffering pain) does so with an air of confidence and of sympathy. In the case of children a hug, a little comforting, and the giving of a portion of an aspirin tablet with great ceremony will very quickly get rid of most minor headaches and all that goes with them. Difficult though it is to believe, do remember that minor pains in four out of ten *adults* are relieved if they are given a simple sugar tablet by someone who appears to be brim-full of confidence in it. So how easy it must be to make children's fears vanish with the pain that caused them! But remember to crush the aspirin in milk or fruit juice; and not to give aspirin to a young child except on a doctor's advice.

Second tip: do bear in mind that a small proportion of people, perhaps 10 per cent of us, probably are more sensitive to pain than the rest; and another 10 per cent are a good deal less sensitive. The more sensitive 10 per cent are not neurotic and they are not malingerers – they really do feel pain more than you and I, and allowance must be made for them.

Third, remember what was said in connection with aspirin: that patent medicine analgesics are usually no good for abdominal pains – indigestion, colic, griping pains. This is because the substances in them simply do not operate on such pains. If a griping pain (apart from period pains in women) does not vanish fairly quickly, consult your doctor. Do *not* take an aperient.

And a final tip in connection with rheumatism, the English disease. Rheumatism that's causing anything more than a middle-aged twinge or two should, of course, take you to your doctor. Sometimes he'll prescribe the cortisone type of drug, or a course of injections; but more often he'll advise pain-relieving tablets, often of the aspirin type. Well now, as he will confirm, it's a good idea to keep the aspirin tablets *and* some water by your bedside, and to take your first dose as soon as you wake in the morning. Then, if you can afford the time, stay in your warm bed for three-quarters of an hour, by which time the tablets will be working fully and you'll find getting up and about much easier.

And which patent medicine analgesic should you use for minor aches and pains? As you will perhaps have realized by now, this book is not intended to lay down the law. It is meant to enable you to decide which patent medicines, if any, are best for your purpose. All one can say in general terms is: be careful with those containing phenacetin, remember that aspirin is the best analgesic of all; and once you've found an analgesic that suits you, stick to it.

And the analgesics in powder form that are popular in the North of England and in Scotland? You will remember the advice always to crush an aspirin tablet into powder before taking it. This is because powdered aspirin is probably a little kinder to the stomach than an aspirin tablet. However, this superiority does not mean that analgesics in powder form should be taken neat – in Scotland some people have a bad habit of shovelling a headache powder straight off the paper wrapping into their mouths. It's a bad habit because any medicine containing aspirin – and practically all these powdered analgesics do – should always be taken with milk or water, if not with a meal.

Why doesn't some enterprising manufacturer make a liquid aspirin? Because, if it's kept in water for more than a day or two, aspirin starts to decompose and releases acetic acid, which gives it a vinegary smell. This sometimes happens when moisture gets into a bottle of aspirin tablets.

And which tablet *does* act faster? Soluble aspirin (the fizzy kind) gets into the blood more quickly than other aspirins, though there are one or two other kinds of aspirin that aren't far behind for speed. Ordinary plain aspirin is relatively slow, but only relatively. This matter of speed could conceivably be of some importance when quick relief is wanted for a headache, but it's of no consequence when someone is taking aspirin over a period for rheumatism. However, anyone who is taking aspirin regularly over a period should be doing so because his or her doctor has ordered it, and so will be taking the kind of aspirin the doctor has prescribed.

And now, if you've developed a headache from trying to absorb all this information, you should at least know what to do.

6

Antacids and Indigestion

THE ACID IN your stomach could burn a hole in a carpet.
This was what the advertisements for one indigestion remedy
used to say some years ago, the implication being that it would
burn a hole in you if you didn't watch out. Actually your
stomach acid could burn a hole in pretty well anything if it
were a little more concentrated. There's certainly enough of it
– the human stomach turns out some five pints of acid juice
every day. And the acid is hydrochloric acid. Quite often, of
course, we need every drop of those five pints – the food items
some British hotels ask our stomachs to digest being every bit
as tough as small carpets. They resemble them in other ways
too.

Seriously, if you think of the foods we regularly put into
ourselves, it is remarkable that the digestive juices of our
stomachs and intestines do manage to break them down into
material our bodies can absorb and make use of. Think of the
kipper and kidneys and kedgeree we have for breakfast (some
of us), the tough steaks and sprouts and sausages we'll eat for
lunch, the nutty fruit cake we'll scoff for tea, the cheese and
celery with which we perhaps finish our supper. All these items
go into that same delicate receptacle just above our navel, and
an hour or two later, having been squeezed and squashed and
partly digested in the stomach, they're passed on to the intestines, which finish the job. And the next day they're part of
one's fingers and toes – that kipper and those sprouts and that
nutty fruit cake. An incredible consummation.

But then the stomach is a remarkable organ altogether. If
one pauses to consider it, one can't but be amazed by the mere

thought of each of us going around with a medium-sized, self-filling bag of acid inside us: babies, Olympic runners, beauty queens, and duchesses. And each of these stomachs is busy all the time, dealing with the last meal or getting ready to deal with the next one. (It really does get ready in advance, for the most powerful stimulus to the production of gastric juice is the sight and smell of a meal.)

However, perhaps the most remarkable thing about the stomach is that it doesn't normally digest itself. Have you never thought about this? Obviously it ought to. Put the stomach of another animal inside yours, as you do when you eat tripe, and it'll be digested in no time at all. So why doesn't one's stomach digest itself, and gradually vanish like the Cheshire Cat's grin? The short answer is that nobody knows for certain. Probably the layer of sticky mucus that covers the lining of the stomach protects it against its own powerful juices, and there are one or two substances actually in the lining that may neutralize the juice. Whatever the reason, the only time that the stomach does start to digest itself is when one has a peptic ulcer.

An ulcer is a break in any of the body surfaces: when we graze ourselves and some skin is scraped off, we have a kind of ulcer. A peptic ulcer can be a gastric ulcer (that is, an ulcer in the stomach, or *gaster*) or a duodenal ulcer (that is, an ulcer in the duodenum, the first part of the intestines, joined to the stomach). It's called a 'peptic' ulcer because it's due, not merely to the acid in the stomach juice, but to a special substance the juice contains, called pepsin, the normal job of which is to help digest the protein foods we eat – the meat and eggs and fish and cheese. However, in the case of someone with a peptic ulcer the protein it starts to digest is that of the wall of the stomach or duodenum; and as a result some of the lining of the wall is eaten away, and an ulcer is formed. The ulcer is round, about three-quarters of an inch across on average, and perhaps half an inch deep.

However, this chapter is not going to be all about peptic ulcers. The information in that last paragraph is just enough to dispel certain odd ideas some people have about them, and to convince the reader that they are serious things to have. Not that there aren't plenty of interesting questions concerning peptic ulcers, but we shan't answer them here because this book is about medicines you can buy at any chemist's for self-treatment, and peptic ulcers should never be self-treated. They should be diagnosed and treated by a doctor.

All this is not to say that the indigestion remedies you can buy at the chemist's are not perfectly sound remedies, most of them. They contain antacids – substances which neutralize acids – and so they *will* neutralize stomach acid, they *will* relieve peptic ulcer pain, and they *will make* someone with an ulcer feel better. And that is one reason why they shouldn't be self-administered by people who think they have a peptic ulcer: they can lead to a false sense of security.

Quite apart from that, how can a lay person be sure he has a peptic ulcer, and not some other condition, needing quite different treatment? Often a doctor will need X-ray films, and will ask for various special tests to be carried out, before he can say a patient has a gastric or duodenal ulcer. Moreover, when he *is* sure, he knows very well that the treatment of a peptic ulcer does not consist simply in giving the patient antacids. Indeed, antacids, while they relieve symptoms, do not apparently help the ulcer to heal at all. (But rest, no smoking, and one ethical drug do.) And lastly, there can be all sorts of complications of a peptic ulcer, calling for special treatment that no one but a doctor can provide. The only safe rule is: if you have any indigestion lasting more than two or three days at most, go and see your doctor. And the indigestion certainly needn't be there all the time for you to start taking it seriously: peptic ulcer indigestion often comes and goes in relation to meals, and may vanish altogether for months at a time.

Some of you are probably saying that doctors are always thinking they're the only people who know anything about health and sickness, and wanting to keep it all to themselves. In fact, there is a great shortage of family doctors today, so that they have far too much work to do. No doctor, however, is so busy that he would sooner you treated a chronic indigestion yourself than came to see him for ten minutes. Properly treated in the early stages, peptic ulcer is often a comparatively minor condition: wrongly treated over a long period, it can cause death.

But is there any evidence that a lot of people with peptic ulcers *are* treating themselves with patent medicine antacids? Well, the evidence is that any doctor can recall instances of such treatment, taken without medical advice. Also, the amount of over-the-counter antacids sold is a good deal greater than the amount of antacids obtained on doctors' prescriptions, and probably more antacids are taken for peptic ulcers than for all other conditions combined. (This is because a peptic ulcer can last for months or years on and off, and because at one time or another probably some ten per cent of the entire population of this country have an ulcer.) Many ulcers probably do get better without any help from doctors and in people who take a patent medicine antacid. And people ignorant of Mont Blanc *have* climbed it safely by themselves.

The manufacturers of patent medicines, however, can hardly be blamed because some peptic ulcer patients treat themselves with patent medicines. They're not angels, but the code that governs their advertising forbids them to recommend their products for gastric or duodenal ulcers, and on the whole they abide by it – if only for safety's sake. Nevertheless, if an advertisement says your product is good for indigestion or acidity, someone with a peptic ulcer is bound to think it will suit him – and he'll start using it. Are you to blame? No more than when someone with a fractured skull decides to take your aspirin tablet because you had recommended it for headache, and he has a headache.

But now what kinds of indigestion *is* it safe to use a patent medicine antacid for? The answer is those common, minor kinds of indigestion that last for a few hours, or at the very most a couple of days, their cause being usually well known to the sufferer. Medically they are due to an acute gastritis – that is, an inflamed, upset stomach. Drinking too much alcohol at a party can cause this kind of indigestion. So can worry and frustration. So can eating too much, or eating some unusual food; and often the victim will have been smoking too much at last night's party as well.

The victim complains of stomach discomfort, vomiting, loss of appetite, nausea, and heartburn; but he will nearly always get better fairly soon without any treatment – though more quickly if he rests and takes nothing by mouth for a time (particularly no alcohol, or tea, or coffee), and later takes a light, milky diet. An antacid preparation (plus rest, etc.) will often relieve the symptoms of such a simple indigestion even more quickly again; and it does so because the irritated stomach has been producing an excess of acid, which has prevented the stomach emptying itself into the intestine. Once the antacid is taken, and this acid is neutralized, the valve at the lower end of the stomach opens, the stomach contents pass through – and the patient feels better. In addition, many antacids release carbon dioxide gas when they come into contact with stomach acid, and the bringing up of this 'wind' seems to relieve the patient.

Before we discuss individual antacids we should say a little about one symptom that antacids almost invariably do relieve – heartburn. This is a burning sensation felt at the bottom end of the breast bone, and it has nothing to do with the heart. (Wind 'around the heart' has nothing to do with the heart either: it's simply stomach wind, which *must* be near the heart because the stomach is near the heart.) Heartburn arises, in fact, at the lower end of the oesophagus (or gullet) just before this joins the stomach, and is due to the presence in the oesophagus of stomach acid. One might think the burning was simply due to irritation by the acid of the lining of the oesophagus, in the same way as acid on the skin causes irritation; but it's now believed to be due to a spasm of the muscle in the wall of the gullet, brought on by the presence of the acid.

Anyway, heartburn is nearly always relieved, as one would expect, by antacids. (Most women with families will know that it's a common symptom in pregnancy, and is then certainly relieved by them.) This straightforward relief is fine if the heartburn is due to a simple indigestion. It can, however, be one of the symptoms of a peptic ulcer and of other conditions; it is the chief symptom – often at its worst when the patient stoops or lies down in bed – in another condition, called hiatus hernia, in which a part of the stomach slides up into the chest. This condition, like a peptic ulcer, can be diagnosed with certainty only by a doctor, and it should be treated by one too. So if you have any heartburn lasting more than a day or two, go and see your family physician.

Well now, having said that you should prescribe over-the-counter antacids for yourself only if you have a simple indigestion lasting not more than a couple of days, what can we say about the antacid substances themselves? What are they? How do they act? What are their snags?

Antacids act by chemically neutralizing the hydrochloric acid of the gastric juice, sometimes with the production of carbon dioxide gas. (Some of them also absorb, or 'mop up', acid and pepsin.) It is because they neutralize acid that heartburn, and stomach pain or discomfort, and spasm of the stomach muscles are all relieved by them. One very well-known antacid, a constituent of various patent medicines, is bicarbonate of soda, or cooking soda, which certainly produces plenty of carbon dioxide gas in the stomach. Indeed, much of the relief it brings is said to be tied up with the burping of it. Bicarbonate of soda is a perfectly good antacid, and quite safe if used only for a short time. It can, however, be absorbed into the body, and so, if taken very often over a longish period, can cause a condition known as alkalosis.

It used to be thought that the carbon dioxide gas released from bicarbonate of soda in the stomach stimulated the production of more stomach acid, so that, in the long run, the patient was worse off than before; but this, doctors now realize, is not true. Bicarbonate of soda has three big advantages: it acts very quickly; it is still kept for cooking purposes in many households, and so is always to hand; and it is cheap.

This is probably the right place for one further note of

caution about indigestion: fizzy aspirin preparations should
not be used for treating it. Such preparations usually contain,
as well as aspirin, some citric acid plus sodium bicarbonate or
calcium carbonate. In water they form citrate and carbon
dioxide gas, which causes the fizz; and a further reaction, involving the aspirin, then takes place. Any surplus citrate will
certainly act as a mild antacid, just as any surplus carbonate or
bicarbonate will; and most cases of simple indigestion do
need an antacid. However, as we have seen already, aspirin
itself can cause symptoms of stomach irritation, as well as
actual bleeding from the stomach; and so, although aspirin
will relieve any headache associated with the upset stomach,
and the antacid will mop up any excess of acid, the aspirin may
also have this most undesirable gastric irritant effect – in a
patient who is taking the preparation because his stomach is
already upset! So you're best advised not to put aspirin, fizzy
or otherwise, into an upset stomach that is causing indigestion.

Both bicarbonate and citrate are absorbed into the body
(into the blood stream, that is): most of the other antacids are
not. The first of these others is calcium carbonate, or common
chalk, another perfectly good antacid, although it can cause
constipation and can result in chalk balls being formed inside
the intestines. A very little of it is absorbed, but this does no
harm unless a person takes large amounts of calcium carbonate
over a very long period. The constipation chalk can produce is
easily prevented by combining it with antacids that tend to
make the bowels loose; and that means magnesium antacids.
Such a combination is very common in patent medicines for
indigestion, the magnesium antacids used being magnesium
oxide, magnesium carbonate or bicarbonate, magnesium
hydroxide, or magnesium trisilicate.

Of the magnesium antacids magnesium oxide is the most
powerful in neutralizing acid. Indeed, it is the strongest of all
antacids. And the one called magnesium trisilicate, a rather
slow-acting antacid, is often found in doctors' prescriptions, as
well as in at least one patent medicine. Doctors often like to
combine it with another popular prescription antacid, alumin-

ium hydroxide, which, like the calcium antacids, tends to produce constipation. Aluminium hydroxide and magnesium trisilicate together make a very effective antacid combination, and in their action on the bowels they cancel one another out.

Our list would not be complete without a brief mention of bismuth antacids – bismuth carbonate, hydroxide, citrate, and so on. Doctors used to think highly of them as antacids, and believed that they had the extra virtue of forming a protective coating on the stomach lining. In fact, although they can still be found in one or two patent medicines, they are weak antacids, and are not as good at protecting the stomach lining as magnesium trisilicate. Nevertheless 'Bismuth' remains something of a magic word for people who are not doctors.

A few final miscellaneous points. Antacids are best taken in liquid form, but tablets and powders are, of course, more convenient. Antacid tablets should be sucked or chewed. If you look at the formulae of some patent medicine antacids, you will see that now and again a patent medicine contains three or more separate antacid ingredients. Such a medicine will be quite effective as an antacid, but there is no scientific reason at all for having more than one or two antacids in a single preparation. A long list of the names of the ingredients may impress some lay people but it will never impress a doctor.

At least one patent medicine antacid contains, as well as antacid ingredients, a substance of a special kind, which acts on the stomach nerves, reducing the amount of acid produced by the stomach and relaxing spasm of the stomach muscle. However, the value of such 'anti-cholinergic' substances is not yet fully accepted by doctors. In addition, some patent medicine antacids contain, as well as their antacids, substances with names like pancreatin, pepsin, and ol. menth. pip.; and we'll deal with all of these in our next chapter.

7

Bad Breath, Poor Appetite, Enzymes, Liverishness, Wind, Diarrhoea, and Piles

IN THE LAST chapter we dealt with indigestion and with the antacids that are used in its treatment. In the two chapters that follow this one we shall concentrate on the other end of the digestive tube, dealing with the equally big subject of constipation and laxatives. But in the present chapter we shall be dealing with remedies for a miscellaneous collection of minor ailments that have only one thing in common – they are all concerned with the digestive system in some way. Minor but not unimportant: wind, for instance, may not kill people, but it can make their lives quite unpleasant.

Well then, first and briefly, halitosis. It can have half a dozen causes – bad teeth, diseased tonsils, and sinus trouble, as well as various disorders of the stomach and chest. Obviously, therefore, the right way to deal with bad breath is to find the cause and then treat it accordingly; and this can be done only by a doctor. Merely to try to suppress the effect without tackling the cause is a poor approach. Whether chlorophyll has any effect on halitosis has not been proved; while the use of antiseptic mouth washes or toothpastes is like saying 'Tut-tut' to a high-powered compost heap. If you suffer from this complaint, go and see your doctor. And don't be shy: he is used to dealing with things a great deal more unpleasant than your bad breath.

Next, the appetite. Most of us these days are concerned with reducing it, and so reducing our weight; and therefore we shall deal in Chapter 10 with drugs that cut down an excessive appetite. Sometimes, however, we suffer from a loss of appetite. This may be because we have an acute illness or are sickening for one; and in that case we should abide by the wisdom of the body, and eat nothing or very little. Chronic illness causing loss of appetite should be dealt with by a doctor. An even more common cause of a temporary loss of appetite, however, is worry, excess of work, or exhaustion; and a good remedy is a glass of sherry before the meal, which will relax our jangled nerves and stimulate the stomach juices.

But are there no alternatives to sherry or a cocktail? Yes, there are some substances called bitters, which for generations have been used in various parts of the world to improve the appetite and digestion. (The pink element in pink gin consists largely of bitters.) There is very little scientific evidence that they do have any effect on appetite, but in view of their widespread use they should probably be given the benefit of the doubt. They are harmless (though some of them are dissolved in alcohol, which will, of course, stimulate the appetite in much the same way as a glass of sherry does); and they have names around which a great romantic poem could be written – gentian, quassia, berberine, calumba, and condurango, picrorhiza, nux vomica, cusparia, serpentary, simaruba, and tinospora. There is also a bitter in dandelion root called taraxacum, and another in hops, called lupulus.

For some reason difficult to fathom the bitters have been relatively neglected by patent medicine manufacturers. There are far more aperients and cough medicines and headache remedies than we need, but few *simple* appetite restorers. Bitters are sometimes found in patent medicines mixed with other substances. For instance, as we shall see later, they are mixed with nerve 'foods' in certain tonics, and are present also in some tonic wines. One particularly absurd combination is that of a bitter with an aperient: the bitter might make a person start eating some good meals, but then the aperient would be giving him a brisk purge – presumably to get rid of all that rich food the bitter had made him eat. ...

However, after the bitters, let us look at the so-called 'digest-ants'. We mentioned, when discussing indigestion, that the food we eat is broken down in the stomach and intestines be-fore being absorbed into the body to be used for building up our tissues, providing energy, and so on. The breaking-down is done by very small amounts of substances called enzymes. If you think of them as rather like the yeast used in making bread, you won't be far wrong. In the stomach there is that enzyme called pepsin, and in the small intestine there is a collection of enzymes from the pancreas (or sweetbread), known as pan-creatin. These enzymes are produced automatically and regu-larly – as regularly as the dawn and the sunset. If, as does occasionally happen, our stomachs cease to produce pepsin, that isn't very important in itself, for everything that pepsin does to food can be done just as well by pancreatin. Occasionally disease of the pancreas may result in the supply of pancreatin giving out, which *is* important; but then such a disease is itself serious and would take us to our doctor anyway.

What certainly does not happen is that now and again we get short of pepsin or pancreatin for a day or two, and as a result suffer from indigestion, wind, constipation, and so on. Nevertheless some antacid remedies for indigestion contain small amounts of pepsin, pancreatin, or another enzyme, called diastase. Though they do no harm, these enzymes can hardly do any good. Indeed, to take them for indigestion is rather like trying to start a car with the help of a torch battery when the car's own battery is perfectly all right but there's a block in the petrol feed. And the position becomes even sillier when, as happens in some products, pancreatin is not given a special protective coating; for it will then be very efficiently destroyed in the stomach by stomach pepsin: the enzymes it contains happen to be proteins, and pepsin's job is to digest proteins.

Of course, in fairness one must remember that those antacid medicines that contain enzymes do also contain antacids, and will therefore relieve many cases of indigestion. The enzymes won't interfere with the antacid effect. And then doctors themselves used to believe that people were quite often short of enzymes, and used to prescribe them quite freely. What probably happened was that these enzyme-antacid products were developed many years ago on the basis of the best medical thinking of the time; and nobody has got around to telling the manufacturers that their products are now very much out of date. This is a common phenomenon in the field of patent medicines, the manufacturers being usually twenty or thirty years behind the doctors in their thinking; and later on in this book we shall see why.

If he thinks his way down the digestive canal (the long tube leading from the mouth to the anus), the first organ a doctor will call to mind after the stomach and pancreas is the liver. Non-medical people are often surprised to hear that the liver has a lot to do with digestion; but of course, as well as dealing with a mass of absorbed foodstuffs that the blood carries to it from the intestine, the liver manufactures bile, which its gall bladder stores, and later pours into the intestines. ('Gall' is just an old name for bile.) It is the colouring matter of the bile that makes our motions brown (and that makes us brown instead if the flow is obstructed, as in jaundice), and certain salts in the bile are essential to the proper digestion of fat.

Because of the many duties it has to perform (some of them unconnected with digestion), the liver is a very complicated and vulnerable organ – perhaps, indeed, second only to the brain in these respects. And so any disease of the liver is fairly serious and should certainly be treated by a doctor. Most people, however, believe that the liver has days when it is slightly off-colour. They feel liverish, they say. They'll be all right by tomorrow. They'll just take a dose of .... And, of course, the drug manufacturers being businessmen and sharing the hotch-potch of ideas about health that most people have got in their heads, there are plenty of patent medicines available for people who are feeling out of sorts, and who think their livers are to blame.

Now doctors don't share this view that the liver is often

subject to minor ailments, lasting a day or so, and easily treated at home. And they certainly don't believe that the patent medicines put out for liver complaints will do any good to the liver, or indeed much good to any other part of the human body. All of them contain laxatives, and so, if in fact the patient is suffering from constipation, some benefit might be gained from taking a dose of these medicines. However, once you have read the next chapter you will realize that laxatives are usually not the right answer to constipation, and in any case constipation has rarely got anything to do with the liver. Also, the laxatives these particular products contain are usually of the strongest, most undesirable kind – jalap, colocynth, scammony, ipomoea, podophyllum: there is no need at all for such powerful and unpleasant substances, and there never has been. And in any case, they do not act on the liver.

The other common constituent of these patent medicines for the liver is a small amount of bile salts – sodium taurocholate and sodium glycocholate. Now it is true that, when the flow of bile from the gall bladder into the intestine is obstructed, so that the patient is jaundiced, or when, after an operation, the bile is being drained away to the outside, bile salts by mouth may be most useful. They will help the patient to absorb fats from his food, and in particular the vitamins that are soluble in fat – vitamins A, D, and E. But such a patient will be in bed, very often in hospital, and certainly under a doctor's care. He certainly won't be treating himself at home with a patent medicine bought round the corner. Bile salts can do no good to someone who merely has a mild digestive upset, and that is probably what lies behind most attacks of so-called 'liverishness' – a mild gastritis, which we discussed in the last chapter, being the commonest cause of the upset, and the liver not being involved at all.

And finally, a note of wry comedy: even if the people who take these 'liver' preparations *were* suffering from ailments that did actually affect the liver and that were of a kind bile salts would be good for, most of the preparations they take would be useless – for the simple reason that the amounts of bile salts they contain are extremely small. They might benefit a jaundiced mouse, but a jaundiced man needs a great deal more.

The next condition we have to deal with is very common, and very embarrassing; and some people think it is also very funny. It is wind. Where, for a start, does it come from, the wind in the stomach and intestines? Most of it, let us be quite clear, is swallowed air. Many of us swallow air unconsciously; others know more or less what they're doing, and for them doctors have a special term – aerophagists, which is a long word meaning air swallowers. Adult air swallowers – regular swallowers, that is – are of two kinds: people who have indigestion of some kind, and who swallow air in an attempt to get relief; and people, mostly women, in whom the air swallowing is a neurotic symptom – a symptom of 'nerves', as we say.

Apart from swallowed air, some of the wind man suffers from is gas that seeps into the inside of the stomach and intestines from the blood that flows through the small blood vessels in their walls. And some of it is gas formed on the spot – either carbon dioxide produced when the acid stomach juice meets the bicarbonate in the intestinal or pancreatic juices, or else other gases formed by fermentation of foodstuffs in the intestines.

Wind may cause no symptoms at all, or else a feeling of distension, or else griping. We feel distended when there's a lot of wind inside us that's staying more or less still, and we have griping when the muscle of the intestine is trying to force gas along and out – when the gas is being moved, in other words. As well as being able to produce these symptoms all by itself, wind can make certain other symptoms worse – for instance, heartburn. And then there are the various noises associated with the release of wind, at one end or other of the digestive tube, or with its passage along the gut. Some expert aerophagists can release gas from their stomachs with a most impressive noise.

Babies, especially greedy babies, are said to swallow a lot

of air; which is why it's usual to spend a few minutes 'bringing up the wind' every time a baby's fed. In fact, whether or not wind really causes babies a lot of trouble is undecided, at least as far as the modern doctor is concerned. Certainly a crying baby swallows a lot of air, and may bring this up later – but it is the crying that causes the wind, and not the other way round. Apart from any air they just happen to have swallowed while crying (and then bring up), the reason why babies seem often to be troubled by wind may be that a baby's bowels haven't yet learnt how to move *anything* along smoothly and without getting tied into knots – food, for instance, or waste material, or gas. And nearly always it is the last item that gets the blame. However, if you must 'bring up the wind', the best way is not to put the baby to your shoulder and then slap him hopefully between his shoulder blades, but to sit him on your lap and then bend him forwards over his own *left* knee.

A state of chronic flatulence (that is, when one is aware almost all the time of wind in one's inside) should be treated by a doctor. Most of us, however, suffer from minor degrees of flatulence from time to time and then some simple remedy can be taken. A few drops of oil of peppermint on a lump of sugar is an old household remedy, and there are one or two patent medicines that have oil of peppermint as their main ingredient. Peppermint oil is one of a whole series of substances, called carminatives, that relieve griping and colic, and assist in the expulsion of gas – up or down. Exactly how they do this we are not sure. They probably stimulate the muscle of the stomach and intestines to contract, and to contract smoothly and efficiently – not to tie themselves into knots, as they often do when we have wind inside us.

Most carminatives are what doctors and pharmacists call essential oils, the stronger varieties of which make up the majority of the counter-irritants, which we discussed in Chapter 3 as constituents of rheumatic balms. Like the bitters that we mentioned earlier in this chapter, these essential oils and the fruits and plants from which they are derived have wonderfully romantic names; many of the plants being culinary herbs. Just listen to the names: aniseed, cajuput, cardamom, and nutmeg; cassia, coriander, rosemary, thyme, dill, and chamomile; matricaria, aurantus amara, pimento, and lavender. They *should* be good for one with names like that.

Most of the gripe water for babies contain dill oil (dill is a herb very like fennel), but it would be difficult to say whether this is just traditional or because dill really is best for babies. They also, most of them, contain some bicarbonate, and this might seem curious at first sight because the acid stomach juice will release carbon dioxide gas from the bicarbonate and so add to the wind inside the baby instead of extracting it. In fact, the addition of a little more gas to the stomach of someone who is suffering from wind often seems to start them burping, and they soon bring up the extra wind plus the original. Anyone who's taken a small dose of bicarbonate of soda when suffering from stomach distension will confirm this. (In addition, bicarbonate, as we saw in the last chapter, helps to move the stomach contents onwards.) If the wind that's making the baby cry is in the intestine, and not in the stomach, the carminative in the gripe water will be much more important than that extra gas. It is the carminative that will smooth the wind's onward passage – and Father's return to his nice warm bed.

As well as figuring in gripe waters, carminatives are used in two other kinds of patent medicine – antacids and laxatives. It's obviously sensible to include some peppermint or cardamom in an antacid meant for the treatment of an indigestion, because very often wind goes with indigestion, and it must be brought up. It's less easy to understand why carminatives are very often found in laxatives; but they are – particularly ginger, peppermint, and a special one called oleoresin capsicum, which comes from pepper fruits (the kinds that also give us cayenne pepper, Hungarian paprika, and the chillies we use for pickling). In fact, many laxative substances make the bowel muscle contract very vigorously, and quite often the muscle ties itself into knots, just as it can when trying to get rid of wind. It's sensible, therefore, to include with these laxatives a carminative that will help to prevent such spasm and colic.

Even more sensible, of course, would be to use laxatives that are less vigorous in their action, and that won't cause any colic; or, even better, use no laxatives at all – unless advised to use them by your doctor. However, plenty of people still think a brisk purge is good for them, and the patent medicine manufacturers like to provide something that has a kick to it, as though they were selling a super grade of petrol; and then they get cold feet and add the carminative, which softens the kick a little.

There are two other kinds of substance used for the treatment of wind. One is charcoal, which is available in patent medicine form. It can certainly hold on to a great deal of gas, and is a traditional remedy for flatulence. The other is a silicone. Yes, the kind of substance, more or less, that is included in car and furniture polishes. A special kind of silicone is now contained in certain patent medicines advertised for indigestion with wind. Much of any gas there may be in the stomach and intestines is present as a foam, and what this silicone does is to break down the foam very rapidly. It certainly does this – a doctor can almost see it happen if he uses a gastroscope – but whether it also helps to get *rid* of the gas is not yet fully proved.

Diarrhoea comes next. It's a curious fact that, while there are dozens of patent medicines for indigestion or constipation, there are very few indeed for diarrhoea. And this isn't because diarrhoea is one of those conditions for which manufacturers must not advertise remedies (like cancer or tuberculosis). There are, as we all know, brief episodes of diarrhoea that are not particularly serious, and that can well be treated with some home remedy; as well as the diarrhoea of such serious conditions as dysentery, colitis, or typhoid fever.

Any of the calcium or aluminium antacids mentioned in the last chapter will, in fact, help to get rid of a mild diarrhoea, and bismuth antacids are a traditional remedy (though most doctors have not bothered with bismuth compounds in recent years). Charcoal and kaolin are also traditional. Yes, much the same kaolin as goes into the poultice, though don't try swallowing a kaolin poultice when your bowels are loose – it contains other things beside kaolin. Needless to say, the best thing to do if you have a diarrhoea lasting more than a day or two is to visit your doctor, or ask him to visit you.

And finally, in this stomach and intestinal rag-bag – piles (or haemorrhoids). There is what doctors call an external pile, which, although it can be very painful, usually clears up in a few days. (A hot bath often brings relief, though occasionally an external pile calls for a very small operation.) And there is the common internal kind of pile, which may make its presence known from the bleeding it causes, or may be forced out of the anus when the bowels are being opened. Sometimes it stays out once it's come out. Piles are really varicose veins occurring in the anus, and are probably due to too much straining in the lavatory over a long period, though they also occur commonly in pregnancy. (The anus, by the way, is the last part of the long digestive tube, the end of what we call 'the back passage'. It opens on to the skin.)

There are a good number of patent medicine pile remedies – ointments and suppositories and even one or two kinds of pill. In view of the probable cause of piles, and the fact that, whether or not it causes them, straining at stool certainly makes them worse, it is almost unbelievable that one kind of patent medicine pile pill contains very strong laxatives. Such pills cannot be condemned too strongly. (If someone's piles are so painful that he is afraid to go to the lavatory, and in this way becomes constipated, then he should see his doctor as soon as possible – not take a patent medicine.) Pile ointments at least do no harm, even if they usually do no good: they can't do much good because most piles are internal and not protruding. Pile suppositories *could* be of some limited value. They contain substances intended to relieve pain and itching, to stop bleeding, and to reduce swelling – all perfectly reasonable objects. Their names don't matter.

However, for two reasons, self-treatment for piles is nearly always undesirable. First, some other and more serious disease may be causing the piles, and only a careful examination by a doctor can prove that the patient has simple piles and nothing else. Second, the majority of piles should be treated by injection or operation, and these can be carried out only by a doctor. It is true that sometimes a doctor will decide that no treatment is needed, or that treatment with suppositories, at any rate for a time, will be sufficient; but he is the one able to decide this, not the patient.

A lot of people with piles are afraid to go to their doctors – because of shyness, or because they fear they really have some more serious disease, or because they've heard that patients get a lot of pain after operations for piles. The fact is that they do get *some* pain, but much less than used to be the case a few years ago, and a great deal less pain than chronic piles will cause. And as for serious disease underlying piles – it is only a small minority of patients who turn out to have anything of the kind; and the earlier a serious disease is diagnosed the greater is the chance of a cure being possible.

The manufacturers have themselves agreed to print on pile remedy containers the words, 'Persons who suffer from haemorrhoids are advised to consult a doctor'. And the Independent Television Authority will not allow any television advertising at all for pile remedies. So never continue week after week using patent medicine suppositories for piles. They're of some value, and if for some reason you simply can't get to see your doctor for a few days, then it is permissible to use them; but never put your trust in them and in nothing else.

8

Constipation

MOST OF THE money spent on patent medicine laxatives is wasted money. It is wasted because a lot of the 'constipation' for which laxatives are taken simply does not exist, while much of the remainder should not be treated with laxatives at all. It would be easy to say that this was the fault of the wicked patent medicine manufacturers – easy but unfair, at least to some extent. Their advertisements have certainly helped to keep public misconceptions alive, but what they have said about constipation in those advertisements has, by and large, been what the general public believed or half believed already, and what doctors used to believe until not long since.

Forty-odd years ago a famous London surgeon was preaching that poisons from the large bowel were the cause of innumerable diseases, and he practised in accordance with what he preached – he removed all or part of the bowel from hundreds of patients, most of them grateful. Any surgeon who carried out that kind of operation today for that kind of reason would be regarded by his colleagues as deranged.

What is the truth about constipation? But, first, what are the untruths, what do many non-medical people sincerely but misguidedly believe about it? They believe that everyone should have a frequent, regular bowel action; and that, if someone 'misses' a day (or it may be two), then his bowels should be *made* to work – with a laxative. They believe that constipation produces poisons that cause headache, loss of appetite, fatigue, bad breath, indigestion, and pimples; and that if a person has one or more of these symptoms, then as likely as not constipation of some kind must be present – and must be treated. It is this kind of thinking that makes a lot of people take a laxative regularly every week, or more often; and as what's good for the goose must be good for the gander, and for the goslings, these people consider it their duty to see that the entire family have a regular 'clean-out' as well. They look upon all bowels as enemies to be subdued.

What is it that makes people think like this about one innocent, hard-working part of the body? Probably it all starts in the first few years of life when many mothers (and grandmothers) watch baby's motions as though they were made of gold. Many healthy babies, particularly breast-fed babies, will quite happily have a motion only every three or four days. This is perfectly normal for them, even though, as they get older, they will usually have a motion more often. However, their mothers don't think it normal. They dose baby with fluid magnesia, or whatever other laxative they think is right for babies; they sit baby on the potty six times a day, and are delighted if he 'does it' in the pot. After all, when he does, it's easy to get the nasty stuff out of sight, and out of mind, down the lavatory pan. When he soils his nappy, however, the nasty stuff has to be laboriously removed and the nappy washed – and even then there's often a stain left on it. A nasty stain, of course.

But how can any baby avoid soiling his nappies, or perform to order on the potty? No child can have any proper kind of control of his bowels before the age of fifteen or eighteen months. His nervous system simply isn't properly developed until then; though, of course, if a baby spends an hour every day sitting on a pot, it's inevitable that now and again he will oblige – purely by coincidence, not because he's beginning to learn. He *can't* learn control at that age – but he can begin to learn what mummy feels about nappies and bowels and motions.

This is the beginning of a long process of getting into our heads that anything to do with our bowels is dirty. But, some people will say, the motions obviously are dirty, they smell and they're a nasty brown colour and they're ... well, they're like cow pats and stable manure. My answer is that cow pats in a field will help to make it grow the most wonderful mushrooms, and that I'll accept as much stable manure for my vegetable garden as anyone cares to offer me. As for the colour of the motions, it's the same as that of chocolate, and the smell is very close to that of certain cheeses.

After all, what do our stools consist of? First, food remnants that we can't digest, chiefly the tough fibrous parts of food. Second, dead bacteria – for our bowels are full of bacteria that are very useful indeed to us. Third, bile pigments that cause the brown colour (and they are formed from the blood). Fourth, water. Nothing horrible in it, is there? No, the plain fact is that people who think their stools nasty and dirty do so for the same reason as makes them believe in the virtues of regularity and the dangers of 'missing a day' – because they were brought up to think like that. And, of course, it is very difficult to throw off what one is taught as a child. Just why our bowels and motions have *come* to be considered nasty would need a lot more space to explain; but it's certainly no wonder that many young children will refuse to have their bowels opened when they're feeling angry with Mother, and *will* have a motion when they're feeling kind towards her. Or that later on they come to regard the bowel, its products, and anything to do with it as making up a horrible monster that can be kept under control only by the regular discipline of a good strong laxative.

And now for the truth about the bowels and about constipation. Many people say they must never leave that 'nasty stuff' inside themselves for more than a day or two at a time because there are poisons in it that will make them ill. What do doctors think of this? Well, there are one or two substances in the contents of the large bowel that *could* make one feel ill if they were absorbed into the body; but we now know that these substances are not, in fact, absorbed. The only symptom constipation *sometimes* causes, apart from the sense of discomfort felt in the back passage, is a headache; and this is due, not to poisons, but to a purely mechanical stretching of the bowel by the retained material. How do we know? Because a doctor can produce exactly the same kind of headache in someone by filling up the person's lower bowel with cotton wool.

Today doctors also realize that the frequency of bowel action can vary markedly from one healthy person to another healthy person. Some people will have a motion two or even three times a day. Others will have a motion once a week. Most people come somewhere in between. 'Once a day' is not essential to good health at all; and indeed is much too often for some people, and not often enough for others. However, miss a day (or, even worse, miss two days), or have any of those symptoms mentioned earlier, and if you're bowel-conscious or have a mother or wife who is, you'll have a laxative inside yourself in no time at all.

Again, some reader is probably saying that, if he gets a really bad head or is off his food or feeling run down, a laxative puts him right in no time. No doctor would deny it. If one really believed that chewing a dock leaf (or even a piece of concrete) would relieve a headache, it often would do so. Those symptoms, you see (headache, feeling run down, being off one's food), are often psychological in origin; and so faith, which is also psychological, will cure them, provided the faith is strong enough. This is no criticism of the symptoms or of faith. The symptoms are real enough, and can have many causes. Faith is real enough. It's just a pity for people to have faith in nothing better than a laxative, and a horror of anything as harmless as their bowels.

Another factor to bear in mind is that people who are worried, especially if they're not fully aware of it, often look ill and run down, and they are also often constipated – because the emotions, as we all know, can affect the bowels. However, friends, seeing such a person, say, 'Ah, ha! run down because he's constipated' – when the truth is that worry lies at the root of both troubles.

But now the person who has got rid of his motion with a laxative, and of his symptoms because of faith in the laxative – what else have doctors got to say about him? Well, a *normal* bowel action empties only the lower half of the large bowel; so before long – in twenty-four hours if your bowels usually act once a day – we shall probably have another bowel action. Not so after a laxative. Doctors know that the *entire* large bowel is emptied by most laxatives; so after a purge the bowel won't trouble us at all for two or three days. There's nothing there, so why should the bowel do anything but have a rest? That's not constipation, it's perfectly natural. And yet the laxative taker will argue that it means he needs another dose of laxative, that he has a stubborn bowel; and on the very day when it would probably have started to function normally again if it had been left to itself, the bowel will be forced into activity again. If it's a young person that's involved, the laxative habit is beginning to be formed, and very soon the bowel will be regularly flogged into activity, and after a time it will cease to work at all unless stimulated yet again by another 'dose'. It's hard by that time to say which is more addicted to laxatives – the bowel or its owner. But the treatment is obvious: to wean oneself off laxatives over a period.

By now it should be clear what was meant at the beginning by the non-existent 'constipation' for which laxatives are taken. Such constipation is simply an absence of bowel action for a day or two, which results either from the bowel having been completely emptied by a previous laxative or from the fact that the bowel of the person in question acts, quite naturally and healthily, only every two or three days and not every day or oftener.

But then what *is* meant by constipation? One is constipated if one starts to have one's bowels opened less frequently than usual or if one's motions are hard and dry. Usually the two things go together, but not always. And much the commonest kind of constipation is not due to any wickedness on the part of the bowel but to carelessness on the part of its owner. Failure to respond to a call of nature is the commonest cause of constipation.

The lowest part of the bowel, called the rectum, is normally empty. It is when the rectum fills up with waste material that we feel the need to empty our bowels; and this normally occurs shortly after breakfast. The taking of food into the stomach at breakfast time – or even the taking of a first cup of hot tea or coffee – is a signal for the next-to-last part of the bowel to empty its contents into the rectum. And suddenly we feel we should go to the lavatory. If we do go and spend five minutes there, then we shall have a motion. In part, this is automatic; in part it's brought about by straining. And, as we've mentioned, when one does have a motion about half of the entire large bowel is emptied of waste matter.

However, suppose we refuse to listen. Suppose we do not go to the lavatory – because we're late and have a bus or train to catch, or because we're just lazy, or because we're angry with Mum. The rectum still becomes full of waste material, which will get dry and hard during the day. If we go to the lavatory the same evening, or the next day, we'll find we have a consti-pated motion. And if we do this kind of thing regularly, per-haps having our bowels opened in the lavatory at the office at eleven o'clock in the morning or at four in the afternoon – not every day, but two or three times a week, when we happen to remember – then we shall get into a state of chronic constipa-tion. Soon the rectum will have waste material in it most of the time. We shall find we cannot recognize a call of nature when we hear one, we've been ignoring the call for so long. And we'll find the rectum and bowel are so lack-lustre we have to take a laxative in order to obtain a worth-while motion. 'Once a week' laxative takers are legion.

This is, in fact, the kind of constipation mentioned at the start of the chapter that should not be treated with laxatives at all. How it should be treated is pretty obvious. Anyone suffer-ing from this kind of constipation should make a resolution that in future he will *always* respond to a call of nature. He should set aside five or ten minutes each day after breakfast for a visit to the lavatory, for it's then the call usually comes. He should sit in the lavatory in peace and quiet, reading if he wants to. He shouldn't worry if nothing happens. He should make sure he's getting the right kind of diet, with plenty of

CONSTIPATION   89

fruit and vegetable in it; and at least four pints of fluid every
day. (The *wrong* kind of diet alone can cause a true constipation.) In this way he'll find that, if he's been taking a laxative
regularly, he'll be able to manage with a milder one taken in-
frequently; and then in smaller and smaller doses – until, in
the space of a few weeks or months, he's able to wean himself
off laxatives altogether. And much the same routine should
be followed by the very frequent laxative taker, whom we
discussed earlier.

But then, is there *no* kind of constipation that calls for a
laxative? And what about the laxatives patients are nearly
always given in hospital? Yes, one is usually given a laxative
before an operation, and before an X-ray film of the abdomen is taken. This is to make absolutely sure that the bowel is
emptied – the patient might be one of those people we've just
described who take no notice of an ordinary call of nature,
and in any case the change of diet in hospital, and fear, and the
strange lavatory may result in constipation. Very often too one
is given a laxative after an operation, or after childbirth. (And
now and again, if truth be told, one is given an unnecessary
laxative in hospital – by a stern and well-meaning sister, who
was taught when she was a probationer nurse. . . .)

What we have been saying about constipation in hospital
leads us to what is probably the commonest of all causes of
constipation, apart from laziness. Any change or upset at all –
an operation, a change of diet or of house, a fever, a day or two
in bed – can lead to constipation. Most of us have experienced
this kind of constipation when on holiday; and, of course, as
soon as our diet returns to normal, or we get used to the new,
strange lavatory in our hotel or boarding house, so soon do our
bowels start functioning properly again. Sometimes on such
occasions a single dose of a mild laxative may be needed.
Usually, however, our bowels settle down just as soon as we
do.

There is another kind of constipation that occurs commonly
in old people. It's very like the sort that results from neglecting
the calls of nature, but in addition the muscles of the bowel

D.Y.T.—5

are weakened in these old people, so that they do need a laxative now and again, as well as some straightforward advice. Old people can also suffer from a peculiar type of constipation in which they pass fluid motions. This is because masses of waste have collected in the lower bowel as we described earlier, and the irritation they cause results in fluid material being passed. This condition calls for attention from a doctor. And so does a condition that doctors call spastic constipation, in which disturbed emotions lead to disturbed motions. And so, of course, does any constipation that comes on suddenly without obvious cause at any age. It may be a sign of a sudden serious block in the bowel, or even of an appendicitis. So never give a laxative in such circumstances, and especially not if the patient has colicky pain. Instead, ask your doctor to come and see the patient as soon as possible. He should also be consulted about constipation of *slow* onset, unless it is due to laziness.

It's a good rule never to give a laxative if you're in any doubt as to whether or not you should. Doctors themselves are prescribing laxatives less and less often. Apart from cases of poisoning and patients who have been given a deworming medicine (in both instances a brisk purge is nearly always desirable), doctors will give laxatives only in some of the special circumstances we've been discussing – to old people, to people suffering from a few days of mild constipation due to a change in diet, etc., and to certain patients in hospital. For instance, although it is traditional to give purgatives to a patient with a fever, most doctors do not now do so routinely. They know that prolonged or excessive taking of laxatives can result in a chronic inflammation of the lower bowel, and in various serious symptoms due to an excessive loss from the body of a mineral called potassium. And if you want even more reasons for not getting into the laxative habit, remember that stopping laxatives after someone's been taking them for a long period may result – for a short time, at any rate – in headaches, giddiness, and loss of appetite. Much better never to start. And never, never take a laxative – or give one to a child – to *prevent* constipation or to 'keep the bowel in order'.

People often ask what is the difference between an aperient, a laxative, and a purgative; and the answer is that, strictly speaking, an aperient is very mild in action, and a purgative is very drastic. However, in practice, the three terms mean much the same thing – a substance that makes the bowels act. There are many such substances, and what they are and how they act we shall consider in the next chapter.

9

Laxatives and Alternatives

DOCTORS USUALLY put laxatives into one of three classes: those that provide bulk for the bowel to act upon, those that are merely lubricants, and those that irritate the bowel and so force it to act.

Of these the substances that provide bulk are the most natural, though still a long way from nature. It is, after all, the sheer bulk of ordinary waste material in the bowel that makes the bowel muscles start the pumping-out action that results in a motion. That is why a first and often effective treatment for an attack of holiday constipation is simply to increase the amount of bulk-producing foodstuffs we eat. In general, apart from plenty of liquid, this means fruit, and root or leafy vegetables: once the body has extracted all their nourishment from them, these do leave a fair amount of roughage. Wholemeal bread is also commonly taken as a bulk provider.

However, if a change in diet doesn't have the desired effect, we may have to obtain extra bulk in some other way. Bran, the substance left when flour is extracted from wheat, provides bulk if taken in *substantial* amounts; but it appears to irritate the bowel in some people. Another bulking agent is agar, or agar-agar as it is often called. Agar is made from Japanese seaweed (although it can also be made from Irish Moss seaweeds), and it swells up when it is placed in water. This is what happens in the bowel: agar greatly increases its own bulk by absorbing water, and so it stimulates the muscles in the bowel wall to become active. Agar is sometimes mixed with other laxatives, though as often as not far too little of it is included to have any worth-while action at all.

A similar substance is methylcellulose, which forms a jelly with water that is ten times as bulky as the original substance; and there are a number of other cellulose compounds that can be used for mild cases of constipation. At a pinch they might also be used for sticking a new wallpaper on the living room walls, for they act as binding agents (like ordinary glue) outside the body, as well as loosening agents inside it.

The other group of substances that will relieve constipation by providing bulk are the saline purgatives – the 'dose of salts' kind. These salts – Epsom salts, Glauber's Salt, and so on – are made up of chemical elements that are not easily absorbed by the bowel in the way that foodstuffs are. Instead, they stay inside the bowel, and, as they pass along it, either draw water from its wall into its cavity, or else, if they are taken with a lot of water, they 'hold on' to this water and prevent it being absorbed. Either way they provide fluid bulk inside the bowel, and this causes the bowel muscle to contract. Salts in solution pass rapidly along the intestine, and so produce a motion in half an hour to two hours; and they are therefore usually taken first thing in the morning on an empty stomach. (The other bulk laxatives are slow-acting.)

Some of the saline purgatives fizz when put into water, and are meant to be taken while still giving off gas. This makes them refreshing and more interesting to take, but makes no difference at all to their laxative action. And, of course, in the case of the well-known Seidlitz Powders (named after a Bohemian village) the contents of the blue and white paper packets, each containing a separate part of the powders, are meant to be mixed in water before being swallowed: don't take the contents of the blue packet, and then the contents of the white one, or you'll have a miniature explosion in your stomach. The fizz, by the way, in these purgatives comes simply from bicarbonate of soda and a weak acid, which act upon one another in water to give carbon dioxide, the gas one finds in any fizzy drink.

Saline purges are popular and comparatively harmless. They're usually taken soon after getting up, and then often in such small quantities that it must be the large volume of water they're taken in that does the trick – that and the small business of measuring out the dose, adding the water, and rinsing the glass, all of which lead the lady or gentleman in the dressing gown to expect a bowel action before long. Expectations of that kind, if they're strong enough, are usually fufilled.

And finally, before we leave the saline purges: the various magnesia preparations that are given to babies and young children for their laxative effect are essentially saline purges. They're also wasted purges very often, because babies and young children, even more than the rest of us, do not commonly suffer from constipation; and when they do, it's usually – at any rate in babies – the result of under-feeding, and should therefore be treated by increasing the size of the feeds.

The second big class of laxatives is the lubricant class, and its only important member is liquid paraffin. Various vegetable oils, like olive oil, have been used as lubricant laxatives but most of any such oil is, of course, absorbed into the body like any other foodstuff, and so they have to be taken in quite large amounts before enough will pass on into the lower bowel to give a worth-while lubricant action. Liquid paraffin, however, is mostly unabsorbed, and is certainly of value where the motions are small, and hard, and dried up, as well as in people suffering from attacks of piles or fissures, or who have had operations on the anus. It is also very popular with old people and expectant mothers. It should be taken between meals, not immediately after one.

Although it is always said to act simply as a lubricant, liquid paraffin may, in fact, stimulate the bowel muscle very gently in the same way as the bulk laxatives do. Altogether, indeed, liquid paraffin is not as innocent and simple as it seems. It is a fat, and so it can interfere with the absorption by the body of those vitamins that are soluble in fat, the most important of these being vitamins A and D. It can 'go down the wrong way' in children and old people, and end up in the lungs where it causes an inflammation. And although it's said not to be absorbed, a little of it can, in fact, pass through the wall of the intestine (or bowel), and will then be carried to some glands in the abdomen, where it gives rise to small paraffin tumours. These are not dangerous. Perhaps the worst fault of liquid paraffin is that – particularly if taken last thing at night in big doses – it can leak slowly from the back passage, and so make a mess of one's underclothing. The taking of small doses, three or four times a day between meals, may prevent this.

On the whole, therefore, quite apart from the fact that very few people truly need a regular laxative, liquid paraffin is not something to be taken day after day, week after week. However, many old people do take a tablespoonful once or twice a week. They get used to it, just as they sometimes get used to a regular dose of Epsom salts or cascara; and it's probably best not to try to stop such a laxative habit in anyone who's really old, unless it is obviously doing harm. To try and stop it only confuses and upsets an old person, and regular laxatives can't usually do much *extra* harm in someone who's been taking them for years.

And, of course, when there's a laxative habit to be broken in someone who is not old, one should always try to break it gradually. If such a person insists on continuing indefinitely to take something for his or her bowels, remember that the old-fashioned prunes are as good as anything; and properly cooked, *can* be very pleasant to take. Prunes are remarkable in that they not only have a bulking action, like Epsom salts or Glauber's Salt, and a lubricant action, but also an irritant action on the bowel wall – like our next big group of laxatives.

This irritant group contains all the substances that first come to most people's minds when they think of bowels and of laxatives: senna, cascara, jalap, calomel, colocynth. However, there are all kinds of irritant purges, ranging from croton oil, a violent-acting and dangerous substance, to certain senna preparations which are fairly mild in action.

Let us start with a collection of four such irritant laxatives that are mostly not too severe in their effect, and that are still widely used. They are aloes, cascara, rhubarb, and senna, and the various preparations made from them. How do they act? Curiously enough, not by moving down the digestive tube till they reach the bowel and then stimulating it. They all contain a number of substances (of which the chief is called emodin) in a form that is not laxative at all. However, these substances are absorbed into the body, changed so that they *are* laxative, and then sent in the bloodstream to the lower bowel – or colon, as doctors call it. Having reached the colon, they stimulate its muscle to act. All this takes time, so that it is usually six or eight hours after a dose of one of these laxatives before anything happens.

Although they are not violent in their effect, some of these emodin purges can be quite powerful, especially if they're taken in what doctors and pharmacists call their crude form – for example, a senna leaf infusion, or an infusion of rhubarb (which isn't the rhubarb we eat as a fruit, but a special kind grown in China and Tibet). Because these crude preparations can be strong, they are particularly liable to cause griping. In addition, senna and rhubarb can colour the urine red; and if any of these purges are taken by a nursing mother, the baby may be upset, for the substances in them do come out in the breast milk. Cascara is the gentlest member of the group, and probably the most useful; but there is a new senna preparation that is both reliable and not too violent in action. Members of the group are present in syrup of fig, and are more important than the fig.

The most powerful of the emodin laxatives is aloes (an extract of which is called aloin). Aloes is best not taken during pregnancy. The *British Code of Standards* governing the advertising of patent medicines lays it down that a warning of this kind (about certain laxatives and pregnancy) should not be given in an advertisement lest the medicine in question might be used in an attempt to procure an abortion. And yet women who are wanting one will nearly always know or be able to find out easily enough that a very strong purge *may* cause an abortion, whereas not a few pregnant women, wanting a baby and ignorant of the danger, must be taking a strong purgative every week in all good faith – simply as a purgative. One does not know for certain that any of them have suffered in consequence; but this does seem to be one occasion on which a good intention may have gone badly astray.

The next irritant laxative, phenolphthalein, is one of the most popular of all laxatives, though it's difficult to say why. Perhaps because it has no taste and so can be taken in ways that would be impossible for any of the bitter-tasting laxatives. Perhaps because its action is not too violent. Perhaps because it used to be thought a fairly safe substance. We now know that it does have certain drawbacks, like any laxative. It sometimes causes a skin rash, it can colour the motions red, and it tends to have a prolonged laxative action – sometimes for as long as three or four days. This is because it is absorbed into the body, passed out again in the bile (so reaching the intestine for a second time), is absorbed again, passed out again, and so on. The laxative action of phenolphthalein was first discovered when it was added, for identification purposes, to cheap Hungarian wine at the start of this century; and since then it has been used in dozens of patent medicine laxatives.

Less widely used than phenolphthalein, though its name is much better known, is castor oil, still a favourite for 'clearing out' the bowels when some undesirable foodstuff has been taken. Castor oil itself is not a laxative, but in the first part of the intestine it forms a substance called ricinoleic acid, which is. It should preferably be given on an empty stomach, it acts in two to six hours, and, although powerful in action, it causes little colic. However, it is not pleasant to take. Castor oil is unique among the substances named in this chapter in that it does not figure in any patent medicine; but it is preferable, as a laxative, to some substances that do.

There are a number of other irritant laxatives, which are violent in their action and should never be used, chief among them being jalap, colocynth, scammony, and podophyllum. Except for podophyllum, they act very quickly, and so violently that blood may sometimes be passed from the bowel. There is no need whatsoever to use such drastic purges (although they are still found in quite a large number of patent medicines); and a restriction should be placed on their sale. Even more undesirable, because of the poisoning it can cause – particularly in infants – is calomel.

The irritant laxatives (or stimulant laxatives, as the milder ones might be called) can mostly cause griping, which is due to the muscle of the bowel going into a violent spasm; and because this effect is so common, they are often combined with substances, such as belladonna, peppermint, cardamom, and ginger, which can relieve such spasm. (We discussed such usage of those last three substances – which are carminatives – in Chapter 7.)

Is there nothing new among the laxatives? Yes, there are at least a couple of new products that seem to be an improvement on what we had before: the new senna preparation we've already mentioned – which any pharmacist will provide – and a product containing a substance called bisacodyl, which is related to a laxative substance found in prunes. One very recent and ingenious idea has been to make a suppository that will release a harmless, odourless gas (carbon dioxide) in the bowel. This does seem to be effective in stimulating the bowel, although suppositories are not nearly so popular in this country as they are on the Continent. Some mothers, imagining a baby or young child is constipated, will insert a crude soap suppository into the baby's anus, but this is a harsh, unnecessary, and most undesirable practice that is mentioned here only to be condemned. Use suppositories only if advised to by your doctor.

In the United States of America enemas, administered in the home, seem to be fairly popular as a means of causing a bowel action; but there is no great demand for them in this country, and every reason why this lack of demand should continue.

10

Slimming

'I LOST TEN pounds in no time' – 'I really let myself go: cream at every meal' – 'It sounds disgusting, but I found I just couldn't squeeze into them.' Snatches of this kind of conversation can be heard at any party, any day anywhere in this country. The topic? It is, of course, that of being fat and being slim, and of people's progress from one state to the other. It is a sad comment on our world that, while millions of people in the West are too fat from over-eating (and are suffering because of it), millions of people elsewhere suffer from hunger, and even starvation.

However, this chapter is not going to consist of a sermon preached at fat people. Whether or not such people are ever gluttons in the old-fashioned sinful sense, there is plenty of evidence that sermons do not, in fact, help them to slim. What obese people need – and what I would guess they want – is understanding and a method of slimming based on such understanding. Equally, of course, I do hope no reader thinks there is going to be any support here for the view that it *isn't* food that makes you fat, or that it's all your glands, or that a glass of lemon juice every morning will keep you slim. It won't do anything of the kind, it isn't your glands, and fat certainly does come from food.

This chapter is going to deal with patent medicines that may help one to lose weight; but these must be fitted into the general picture of obesity and slimming, so let us now take a panoramic look at the slimming field. First, why should one slim? The vast majority of people who are obese want to lose some of their fat simply because our society doesn't approve of

fat people. (Just why society doesn't is another and a complicated matter.) In particular, in the case of women, it's a powerful motive that men don't like flirting with or making love to
fat ladies. Not that most women go around expecting, or hop-
ing for, that kind of thing; but they like to think it's always on
the cards. If society didn't frown on fat, I doubt that most
people would bother about it, no matter what doctors said,
even in books.

There are, however, plenty of good *medical* reasons for not
being fat. Most important is the established fact that fat people
die a good deal earlier than people who are not fat. Even quite
a small increase over one's desirable weight can shorten one's
life: an increase of one per cent in death rate for each pound
that one is overweight is a rough guide. This means that, if one
hundred out of a group of people of normal weight were to
die in a given period, then in the same period, out of a group
of the same height and that was exactly the same in all other
ways except that everyone in it was thirty pounds overweight,
130 would die.

Why *would* those extra thirty die? Because a lot of diseases
are commoner in the obese. Diabetes, for instance, and angina
pectoris, bronchitis, high blood pressure, and gall-bladder
diseases. Arthritis too is commoner, and so are varicose veins
and flat feet and certain kinds of skin rash. Fat people are
more prone to accidents. They get backache more often. However, most of them are not deaf, and they've heard all this many
times before and it hasn't made much difference to them.

They've also heard that, if one takes in more energy calories
as food than one gets rid of in exercise and in keeping up the
body's temperature, etc., the surplus calories will become fat
in the body. We now realize that this is probably not the complete truth – some people, for instance, are apparently less able
to burn up surplus calories than others, and ordinary cane
sugar is a more certain fattener than other carbohydrates. (It
may, in addition, help to cause coronary heart disease in men.)
However, the equation, 'Food intake minus energy output

equals extra fat', remains *broadly* true, and is the first thing to be kept in mind by anyone who's overweight. (There is a minority of people whose excess weight is due to muscle, not fat; but it is a very small minority.) Notice that, if people take practically no exercise at all, they may be fat although eating only the same amount of food as normal people. However, most fat people, as compared with others, probably do eat more and take less exercise as well.

There are, of course, good reasons for taking exercise apart from the fact that it does burn up some of one's surplus calories. The best of reasons, and one that doctors sometimes forget to tell their obese patients, is that exercise is enjoyable. It is very easy to forget this now that the motor car and the television set rule our lives; but running and jumping and climbing, and swimming and playing any game you care to mention – all these are pleasurable. Indeed, the idea that exercise is not a matter for enjoyment is a hangover from the time – which ended quite recently – when most of the exercise most people took was the hard manual work they had to indulge in if they were to go on living: banging and hammering and digging, walking miles to work, washing clothes by hand, lifting and tugging and pulling. All that has now finished for most people in the Western world: it is a lack of exercise that is the menace now – not an excess of it.

As for the pleasure of exercise, each of us, after all, has a body made up of bone and muscle that were meant to be used, covered with a skin that was meant to sweat now and again and to have fresh air playing upon it. And we are weak creatures: we'll do things that we like readily enough, and will soon forget about those we don't. So why not make use of this weakness when we can? Choose your favourite form of exercise, and practise and enjoy it every day; though don't at first go in for too much of it if you're overweight.

One important reason for fat people taking exercise, apart from the calories it consumes, is that it may help to regulate our appetites according to what our bodies really need. Thus, if rats are given no exercise, they will eat and eat, and grow fatter and fatter. But if they are given quite a moderate amount of exercise, they eat only enough to keep their weight steady, no matter how much food is offered to them; and most curious of all, no matter how much extra exercise they are given, they will go on adjusting the amount of food they eat to the amount of energy they're expending on the exercise – and their weight will remain steady. The more exercise they take, in other words, the more they eat. Human beings are not rats, of course, but they may react similarly in certain respects.

And now a few words about 'energy'. Many people cannot understand when doctors talk about intake of energy and expenditure of energy. They think of energy as something that children and young people have plenty of, something that shows itself in their jumping about and never getting tired. (The right word would be vitality.) But doctors have an extra meaning for energy – to them it can also mean something that we all get from our food and that keeps our organs and body tissues going in their humdrum everyday physical activities, whatever our age may be; and that also feeds the muscles that enable us to walk along if we're middle-aged, or to hop, skip, and jump if we're young.

The human body is rather like a railway engine: food is its fuel, and what makes *its* wheels go round is the energy it obtains from food, just as the engine obtains energy from coal. Everybody knows what will happen if every day coal is put on a railway engine that is making only a few short, slow journeys, and otherwise is simply supplying hot water for the driver's pots of tea: it will be smothered in coal before long. And that is what happens to the human body when it takes in food supplying more energy than the body is using up.

A calorie is a unit of energy. (A Calorie, with a capital 'C', is a thousand small calories.) And there are no foods worthy of the name that supply no calories or practically no calories. In general terms, the more satisfying a food is, the more energy calories it is supplying. Thus fatty foodstuffs, like butter and cream and chocolates and pork and roast duck, which most people find satisfying and pleasurable to take, supply more calories than any other kind. And foodstuffs like fruit juice or cabbage or cucumber, which are pleasant enough to take, but usually only with other foods and never as a main course for a hungry man – these are low in calories. If it weren't so, if there were plenty of foods that were at once very satisfying and pleasant to take *and* low in calories, then there wouldn't be any fat people: anyone who was beginning to get fat would simply switch to such enjoyable, satisfying, low-calorie foods, and be slim in no time at all.

We have now reached the crux of the slimming problem. Habit aside (although eating habits are very important), most people find eating a very pleasurable, comforting activity, and indeed for some people it may satisfy a deep emotional need. Why do businessmen have so many business lunches? Why do we have special meals at weddings and at funerals? Because, when people are anxious or depressed or involved in most other kinds of emotional upset, they seek relief almost automatically in food and drink. This is the reason why, although it isn't difficult, on almost any reducing diet, to lose weight for a few weeks or even a few months, the great majority of slimmers put the weight back on again in the end. They simply start eating to excess again – partly because it's easy to slip back into old habits, but partly because eating gives them great pleasure and satisfaction and comfort, and sometimes nothing else will. Who can blame them? One may disapprove of their fatness, but it's difficult to be censorious about what led to it.

Once this central truth is appreciated, it is easy to understand that there is no simple answer to the obesity problem. It's not just a question of taking a diet, or a drug, or a course of exercises. It's a question of all these, and of anything else that will help one to keep down one's food intake (including a search for hidden worries and tensions). A global strategy, in other words, with the fat person as the globe.

The very first dietary rule is, of course, to take a low-calorie diet, and that means less food. A new wonder diet appears every six months; but it really makes no great difference whether your diet contains a lot of grated carrot or no bread at all or a pint of banana juice a day – so long as it is low in calories and supplies the body with its essential nourishment. Recently there has been a vogue for a high fat, high protein diet, and certainly such a diet can be more satisfying than others, and it will make one lose a good deal of weight in the first week. In the long run, however, although it may be better than any other kind of diet, it is probably not a great deal better. There is no such thing as a reducing diet on which you will never feel hungry: when your body finds itself short of energy calories, it will start to burn its own fat in order to get some. This is, of course, the aim and object of every reducing diet. And once your body does start to use up its surplus fat you are aware of the fact – and you feel like a meal. You feel hungry.

Probably the best sort of diet is one in which there's a marked or even complete reduction in most carbohydrates (sugar, jams, sweets, cakes, biscuits, pastry, bread, and potatoes) and in alcohol, but in which, apart from that, every one of the normal foods is represented, though in slightly reduced amount. In fact, such a diet will have a fairly high protein and fat content. There are some foods the cutting down of which isn't necessary – lean meat, fish, eggs – but by and large your diet should be a balanced one. That means it should contain a modest portion of most things you normally eat (apart from the carbohydrates and alcohol we mentioned just now). If you take such a diet, you certainly shouldn't need any extra vitamins. Include in your diet as many chewy and crunchy items as you can – they help to allay hunger.

A few extra hints about dieting. Don't go in for miracle slimming foods, because there are no such foods: all foods are fattening, and those that are less fattening than others are nearly always less satisfying as well. Starch-reduced rolls are something of an exception: they provide less starch and more protein than ordinary bread, and so, although they certainly provide some calories, they do fit conveniently into a 'low carbohydrate' diet. However, they will be part of the diet – don't get to thinking you can eat them till the cows come home.

If you do, you'll simply gain weight as you will from any food taken to excess.

When on a diet, don't try to lose more than about a couple of pounds a week at most. Don't think, because you lose five or six pounds very quickly, that you'll be through with this reducing business in no time at all: it's pretty easy for anyone to lose a few pounds quickly, what is lost being mostly fluid. The difficulty is in losing a few more pounds, and above all, in not putting them back once you've lost them: in forming new eating habits, in other words. Don't go in for Turkish baths: they'll sweat a few pounds out of you, just as fluid, and you'll drink it back again in a matter of hours. Don't expect massage, in any form – or any other external application – to do the job for you: it'd take a long time for massage to rub away a ton of coal on that railway engine, wouldn't it? It's the same with the fat around your middle.

If you're very serious about losing weight, or are really obese, or if you're thinking of any diet that means more than just giving up sweets and cakes and biscuits and sugar in your tea, then you should consult your doctor. Let him decide if you're fit to go on a really low-calorie diet for a time, let him decide just how much weight you should aim to lose. He will probably want to ask a few questions about your work and about your life. Why? Because, you will remember, we said earlier that over-eating satisfies an emotional need in many people. Your doctor may be able to put his finger on some tension in your working life, or some disappointment or grief you had almost forgotten about (because it was too painful to keep remembering all the time), but that had been nagging away inside you and making you eat too much. Not everyone who's overweight has a secret sorrow or a hidden worry; but some people have, and you might be one of them. In any case, people find it much easier to stick to a diet if they have someone to whom they can talk freely about their difficulties and temptations, and a sympathetic doctor will always listen.

Another thing your doctor may do – apart from prescribing a diet – is to prescribe a drug that will help you to stick to it.

Now, although a lot of obese people think this is the be-all and end-all of visiting their doctor, he himself will tell you it isn't very important at all. Sometimes he will prescribe a sedative (a nerve-quietening drug) that may be quite helpful in the first few difficult weeks of sticking to a diet. At other times he will prescribe an appetite-reducing drug. We shall not spend much time on drugs of this kind, because this is a book about over-the-counter drugs, and the general public cannot now buy the common appetite-reducing drugs freely. However, for the sake of completeness, let it be said that such drugs, although some-times useful for a few weeks, are rarely of value for longer than that, and nearly all of them are brain-stimulating drugs to which people can become addicted. The well-known purple-heart tablets contained an appetite-reducing drug plus a seda-tive. *Don't* try to nag your doctor into prescribing such a drug for you; and if he should agree one would be suitable, *don't* take it for any longer than your doctor thinks necessary.

And now at last we have reached the patent medicine reduc-ing products. Actually this long introduction was meant to make you see that the very next sentence is a reasonable one. Slimming is a serious business that should usually be super-vised by a doctor; and those drugs that are of some real value (and they aren't many) are available only on a doctor's pre-scription.

However, what kinds of patent medicine reducers are there? First, there are products that consist largely of laxatives. They contain substances like aloes, rhubarb, phenolphthalein, and cascara. If you weigh yourself before and after having a bowel action, you will certainly find that a motion can mean a loss of a pound or two in 'weight'; and the loss can be more after taking a laxative – though most of the increase will be due to water. You won't need to be told that a loss of this kind isn't a true loss of weight at all, and is certainly not a permanent loss: it is simply a loss of waste material (which you'd have lost anyway, sooner or later) or of water (which your body will soon make good). In addition, to go on taking laxatives day after day is most undesirable, and may be dangerous to your health. If you're in any doubt on this topic, read the last two chapters again.

Of course, when one is on a strict reducing diet, one sometimes does get constipated because the diet isn't supplying enough bulk to stimulate the bowels. It's a good thing then to take a *mild* laxative. However, this is quite different from pretending that a laxative itself can produce any true loss of weight. The only way in which it could conceivably do so would be by hurrying food along the intestines so that it could not be absorbed into the body; but only a big dose of a powerful laxative would do this, and it need hardly be said that such an action, experienced day after day, might do very serious harm.

It is difficult not to say of laxative slimming products that they should all be thrown down the nearest drain; and, in fact, the *British Code of Advertising Practice* forbids the advertising of any slimming remedy the use of which might prove harmful, and more specifically the advertising of these laxative slimming preparations.

Such preparations sometimes contain, as well as a laxative, seaweed extracts, presumably for the iodine in them. These can do no good whatsoever to the average obese person, but are presumably included because of the old medical usage of thyroid extract for reducing. The thyroid gland in the neck uses a lot of iodine, and it regulates the rate at which the body burns up its fuel; so that, by giving big doses of thyroid, one can cause a fat person to lose weight – though only at the cost of giving him a lot of very unpleasant symptoms as well. Because of those symptoms, most doctors abandoned the use of thyroid extract years ago. However, iodine itself, even though it is stored in the thyroid gland, will not act like thyroid extract – it won't, in other words, make you lose weight, or have any other effect at all, unless you happen to be short of iodine, which is extremely unlikely.

A second kind of weight-reducing patent medicine contains a substance called methylcellulose, which we discussed in the last chapter; or a similar substance. Methylcellulose is harmless enough. It has the property of 'taking up' water inside the body, and thus swelling to a volume much greater than its original one. When it does this in the intestine, it stimulates the bowel muscle to contract, and so acts as a bulk laxative. When it does it in the stomach, it may deceive the stomach into thinking that, because it seems to be full, a good meal has been had. Actually the stomach is nearly always a great deal wiser than that; and although methylcellulose is of some value in some people who are trying to stick to a diet, the value is only slight. Methylcellulose is available as granules, but it is also a constituent of some powdered reducing 'foods', and of some reducing biscuits, though not always in sufficient amounts to have any worth-while effect. After it has 'deceived' the stomach it will, of course, pass on into the intestine, and act as a laxative; but it has none of the vigorous actions of some of the 'reducing' laxatives we discussed just now.

Those are the only two kinds of weight-reducing patent medicines. However, very similar to patent medicines in the way people regard them are the various reducing foods in powder form – those that supply 900 calories a day in various flavours, and that were very popular a couple of years ago. These foods are really the same as an ordinary reducing diet except that all the individual food ingredients that you would normally be taking in, say, beef and cheese and lettuce are all lumped together into what a lot of people would think a rather uninteresting and rather expensive product. (The manufacturers *hope* all the ingredients are there, though there may be one or two essential ingredients of foodstuffs that science hasn't yet discovered.) There is no doubt that, if you stick religiously to the instructions that go with products of this kind, you will certainly lose weight; and equally there is no doubt that some people have found it easier to stick to these powders than to an ordinary reducing diet. However, you will lose weight on *any* low-calorie diet, so long as you stick to it. Much the same as what we have said about these powders can be said about most of the reducing biscuits.

It has been suggested that the very great success of these

powder products – commercial success, that is – was due to the fact that they took people back to an infantile level of eating – to the early days of life when one lived on milk and slops. Whether or not this is true, it will serve to remind us yet again that many people over-eat for psychological reasons, and that these reasons, when present, must be dealt with if a permanent weight loss is to be obtained. Unlikely though it may seem, there is probably a psychological element in the successes achieved with the latest method of slimming, which consists of medically supervised fasting (often by a number of patients together), followed by a period on a diet. The fast is absolute: patients are allowed to take only water, or else black tea and coffee as well (but, of course, without sugar). And this starvation state is kept up for one or two weeks or even longer. After the fasting period the patients are put on a reduced-calorie diet, but they can have fasts lasting one or two days if they find they are putting on weight again. One of the latest methods is to give the patients a two-day fast to begin with, followed by a diet consisting of six small meals a day instead of three of more normal size. Fasting, of course, should never be practised except under medical supervision.

You may be asking, 'Where is the psychological element in all this?' Well, the method is new, and starvation is exceedingly impressive to anyone; and perhaps even more impressive is the fact that, after the first twenty-four hours of complete fasting, appetite is lost (whereas on the usual reducing diet the patient can feel quite hungry). And then the patients do lose a lot of weight quickly – as much as two and a half pounds a day may be lost, and one pound a day is quite usual. Patients feel they are taking a part in something dramatic and exciting; and that there is, perhaps for the first time, a real chance of them becoming slim and staying slim. All this must have a profound effect in the prevention of back-sliding. It is, of course, similar, this fasting method, to what is practised with some success in one or two health establishments in this country – though these are not run by doctors.

One can probably be sure of two things for the future in

connection with losing weight. One is that new and dramatic methods will be introduced (including new kinds of fasting), so that once people have lost weight they will not quickly put it on again. The other is that patent medicines will have even less part to play in helping people to become slim or to stay slim than they have at the moment.

11

Colds

PEOPLE OFTEN say, 'Isn't there *anything* you can do for a cold, Doctor?' Of course, they don't really expect an answer because everyone has his or her own infallible means of shortening colds – and frequently a means of preventing them as well. And they don't seem to notice the contradiction. As often as not the question is asked only so that the questioner may tell the doctor just how he *ought* to be treating colds in his patients. Alas! the majority of doctors remain unconvinced: they think the biggest part of the treatment of a cold is still the grin you give before you start bearing it.

This, at least, is what the vast majority of doctors will tell one in public. In private, however, quite a few of us indulge in treatments of colds, particularly our own colds, that we would pooh-pooh if suggested by anyone else. To give just one example: there is a little evidence that, if one takes big doses of vitamin C regularly, one will get fewer and shorter colds. And a little evidence that very big doses of vitamin C, taken from the start of a cold, will shorten it. Accordingly, some doctors have faith in vitamin C, particularly in huge doses taken as soon as a cold has started.

The evidence for vitamin C is very far from being convincing, but it is partly a faith in vitamin C that explains the widespread usage of fruit juice products for the prevention and treatment of colds, whether the fruit juice product is taken neat or mixed with a fish liver oil. What else lies behind this usage? First, faith in some substance called bioflavonoids that are often found with vitamin C in nature, and that were thought a few years ago (but not now) to be just the thing for the common cold. Second, and most important, drinks made from such fruit products as lemon juice or blackcurrant jam have been used for centuries in the treatment of the common cold. However, the centuries of use prove absolutely nothing: for thousands of years people believed the world was flat. And is it?

What else *may* help to prevent colds? The fish liver oils we mentioned as being sometimes taken with fruit juices – these oils contain vitamins A and D. We know that a lack of vitamin A (now practically never seen in this country) can affect certain lining membranes of the body, and, therefore, it is argued, as colds affect the lining membrane of the nose, perhaps vitamin A will prevent one getting them. This is a weak argument, and certainly not strong enough to justify, as a preventative of colds, the taking of fish liver oils in big doses.

Some people believe in regular gargles as a means of cold prevention. These gargles usually contain antiseptics, often in small amounts. This, however, is a very reasonable economy, for antiseptics can have little permanent effect on the germs of the throat and nose, whether they're present in a low or a high concentration. Even more reasonable and economical would be not to use a gargle at all. Other people believe in bacterial vaccines, taken by mouth, and the best one can say about these is that their value is unproven, and probably either very small or non-existent. Other people are great believers in cinnamon. Well, we all must have faith in something; and for what it's worth, I was told a few years ago that the men working in one London warehouse containing cinnamon never catch a common cold. *Never*, Doctor.

In case all this sounds too disheartening, here are a few positive recommendations that doctors usually put forward: accepting them will certainly do no harm, even though there's no proof they will do any good, at least in the way of preventing a cold. Take a good mixed diet. Take some exercise every day, preferably in the open air. When colds are about, avoid as far as you can situations that involve you being close to a lot of people: travelling in crowded Tube trains, spending Saturday evening in the cinema, and so on. Avoid stuffy, over-heated atmospheres. And avoid chills. Colds are certainly not caused directly by one getting cold and wet, but a 'chill' *may* conceivably lower one's resistance to infection, so making a cold more likely.

So much for cold prevention. Now what else should we know about colds before getting down to their treatment? Colds are due to infection by a tiny organism called a virus, which reaches one's nose in very small, invisible droplets from the throat or nose of someone who is infected with it. As with any infectious disease, the body learns, during the time it has a cold, how to deal with the virus; and it remembers for quite some time how to deal with that particular virus. However, a number of different viruses can cause a cold, and learning how to deal with one kind won't help if you become infected with another. Certain bacteria, although they do not cause colds, may be important in that they probably follow in the wake of the viruses once the cold is under way, and lead to the thick yellowish nasal discharge that cold sufferers often get after the first two or three days.

Odd though it will seem to many people, there may sometimes be a psychosomatic element in the common cold. There *may* be. In other words, one's emotional state, one's mood, how one is feeling about life, may determine whether or not one falls victim to a cold virus, and may affect the duration and severity of a cold.

All right, so how *should* one treat a cold? Some people think that the very first thing to do is to isolate oneself, preferably in bed, for the first two or three days. They are very uncomfortable days, for one thing; and by spending them in bed one may help to ensure that one's cold lasts only a week, instead of a fortnight. It is a most gratifying thought too, that, by staying in bed, one avoids infecting other people: it gilds the lily of repose with the lacquer of virtue. Alas! Nowadays doctors don't regard colds as particularly infectious. However, if you stay at home, at least your friends and colleagues will be spared the depressing sight of you sneezing and blowing and streaming, and the thought that now they're bound to 'catch it'. Such a thought might conceivably ensure that they do catch it.

It will be helpful, if, as we progress through the wealth of patent medicine remedies there are for colds, we keep firmly in mind that the first and basic element of a cold is swelling and inflammation of the lining membrane of the nose, with the pouring out of watery fluid. Later, as already explained, this often becomes thicker and yellowish. In either case the nose is blocked. Second, there is sometimes a sore throat, and a cough may develop. Third, almost invariably there is a headache and a mild fever, and there may be pains in the limbs or back. Medicines for the cough and sore throat of a cold will be discussed in the next chapter; but those for the nose, and for the fever, etc., will be dealt with here.

One's nose, then, that very unlikely object which takes the brunt of a cold's assault. A number of kinds of remedy are available – drops, nasal sprays, and inhalers, chiefly for the early stages of a cold; and ointments, inhalants, and aerosols for the later stages. Drops are watery or oily fluids, intended to be inserted into the nose, a few drops at a time, with a glass dropper. Nasal sprays have a nozzle which is inserted into each nostril in turn; and when it is in, the other nostril is closed, the body of the spray is given a squeeze, and one inhales simultaneously. Inhalers are hollow tubes, perforated at both ends, and containing a solid stick impregnated with a volatile medicine. They are used in much the same way as the sprays, except that an inhaler can't be squeezed: it's the sniff alone that does the trick. Or, rather, two or three sniffs do it.

Ointments: some are meant to be applied to the lining of the nostrils, others are meant to be applied to the chest. Inhalants are pleasant-smelling fluids, which are inhaled either after being put in a jug of steaming water or directly from a handkerchief or pad on to which the fluid has been emptied. And an aerosol is – well, an aerosol that's meant to be sprayed into the bedroom or living room where the victim is situated.

Those last three kinds of 'local' treatment are best suited to the later stages of a cold when there is thick secretion, although they can be used earlier. The two kinds of ointment usually contain menthol and camphor (cooling and stimulating respectively, and both have an interesting smell), plus pleasant-smelling, mildly antiseptic substances like eucalyptus oil, turpentine oil, thymol, methyl salicylate, and geranium oil. Most of these substances are counter-irritants, the properties of which have already been described in Chapter 3 in connection with rheumatic balms.

Apart from their interesting, antiseptic smell, these various substances don't do much good and they don't do much harm – although they could have an undesirable effect on the lining membrane of the nose, especially if applied too high up in it. When applied to the nostrils, they probably stimulate the nose to produce a watery fluid, and this will help to remove any thick secretion and so to unblock the nasal passages. Also, of course, cold sufferers find the smell very impressive – not surprisingly, as practically no other smell registers with them at all. In the case of ointments meant to be rubbed on the chest, the heat of the body causes the aroma of the various oils to be wafted up to the patient's nose – and indeed, to the nose of anyone who happens to be near him. This can reflexly produce a watery nasal discharge.

Aerosols contain the same or similar ingredients, and are really just a modern form of the inhalants, which are liquids, supplied in bottles or capsules, to be breathed in direct, or in a steam inhalation. Very often these contain much the same ingredients as the ointments, extra substances that are sometimes used being peppermint oil, oil of pine, oil of lavender, and oil of cinnamon (all of them pleasant-smelling essential oils, which we discussed in Chapter 7). Much the oldest and cheapest of the inhalants is Friars' Balsam, one teaspoonful of which is added to a jug of water just off the boil, the resulting medicated steam being inhaled through a funnel made with a towel. The steam, which condenses as droplets in the nose, helps to produce a watery fluid which will wash away any thick secretions. Steam inhalations should, of course, be used with great care, if at all, for children; and ointments containing menthol or camphor should never be applied to the nostrils of a young child – they may cause collapse.

And now for the three kinds of local treatment meant to be used chiefly in the *early* stages of a cold. Practically all nasal drops and sprays, and some of the inhalers, contain substances, called vasoconstrictors, that close down the tiny enlarged blood vessels in the inflamed lining of the nose, and thus reduce the swelling of the lining. As far as the patient is concerned, the effect is to reduce the nasal blockage and dry up the secretion. Among the many substances used for this purpose are ephedrine, phenylephrine, and tetrahydrazoline.

Preparations containing these substances should not be used automatically just because one has a cold, and in any case not for more than a few days. Indeed, some doctors think they should not be used at all. This is because they can interfere with the delicate self-cleansing action of the nasal lining, and because, after the initial shrinking of the nasal lining that they cause, there is often a 'spring-back' with most of them, so that the membrane is even more swollen than at first. In fact, they sometimes prolong a common cold, and even lead to complications. A final criticism of them is that, in any case, their value tends to decrease with repeated usage.

However, it must be admitted that these sprays and drops can be helpful if one simply *has* to fulfil a short social engagement when suffering from a cold (one demanding a speech, for instance); and used with care, they do bring some temporary relief of symptoms to the cold sufferer. A spray, which spreads out on the lining membrane of the nose, is preferable to drops, most of which will just be swallowed straight away. However, of the drops the watery kind is to be preferred to the oily kind. And remember that ephedrine is probably at least as good and as safe as any of the other vasoconstrictors found in these sprays and drops, as well as being cheaper.

Some of the nasal drops contain, as well as substances that close down the small nasal blood vessels, our old friends camphor, menthol, eucalyptol, etc.; and many of the inhalers contain *only* such substances, and no vasoconstricting substances at all.

And now, having dealt with the various local treatments for the nasal congestion caused by a cold, what about a medicine to bring down the fever and relieve any headache and pains in the limbs? The answer, of course, is to take one of the analgesics, or pain-relieving drugs, we considered in Chapters 4 and 5: aspirin, phenacetin, paracetamol, and so on. The best of them is aspirin, which is present in a great many patent medicines, though a standard aspirin tablet, if made by a reputable firm, can be just as good, and cheaper. Sometimes a special kind of analgesic for colds is produced – by adding to the basic analgesic a substance such as menthol or camphor or cinnamon. They have no special advantage over the straightforward analgesics, especially as one cannot smell the extra ingredients in a tablet or capsule that is meant to be swallowed down. Quinine is also added to these preparations on occasion.

But now what about those special cold remedies, the tablets or capsules one takes by mouth that will do simply everything that can be done to a cold? – Short of actually getting rid of it, that is. These products came to us from the U S A a few years ago, and it is pleasant to think that they may have been devised by some tidy-minded pharmacist who himself had a cold and got fed up with all the different things he had to take. Imagine him sitting by the fire, a drink of hot lemon juice (or perhaps a vitamin C tablet) on one side, and a couple of analgesic tablets on the other; and in his hand a spray or a bottle of nasal drops, containing one of those vasoconstrictors we've just been talking about. It's pleasant to think that he suddenly said to himself, 'Eureka! I'll put the whole lot together in one small anti-cold tablet, and that'll be that.' Because this is exactly what was done.

All these products contain a pain and fever reliever, such as phenacetin or paracetamol, perhaps with added caffeine. They all contain a vasoconstrictor such as ephedrine or phenylephrine. And practically all of them contain vitamin C. Are they any good? Well, they're not miracle products. As you might expect, they're about as good as the same ingredients taken separately. However, they're certainly convenient. They also have one snag, like most of the improvements man is hopefully thinking up from his cradle to his grave. When one gives a vasoconstrictor in nasal drops or a spray or inhaler, its effect is more or less confined to the nose. But if one gives it in tablet form, then the tablet is absorbed from the stomach and its ingredients are carried in the bloodstream all over the body and, therefore, act all over the body, not merely in the nose. Vasconstrictors, taken in a tablet, will close down small blood vessels everywhere, and so lead to something of a rise in blood pressure. This is of no great importance in someone who's healthy (though occasionally it is associated with palpitations and 'jitteriness'), but it is undesirable in someone whose blood pressure is already raised or who has a heart ailment. And it could lead to a doctor prescribing more of an anti-blood-pressure drug than a patient needs.

Doctors are still occasionally asked whether antihistamines (the drugs that are of value in case of hay fever) are not effective against the common cold. Some years ago there was a great vogue for antihistamines as cold remedies in the USA, but careful investigation revealed that they are of no value in the true common cold. When a watery nasal discharge is due to an allergy (as hay fever is), and not to a virus infection, antihistamines will certainly be most useful; but most watery nasal discharges outside the hay fever season are not allergic at all, and it's wise to ask your doctor for his opinion if you suspect that yours may be. In any case, antihistamine drugs should be taken only if your doctor advises them or agrees to your taking them. They can, for instance, make you quite drowsy, and they are found in various ethical tablets, sprays, and drops.

Finally, having threaded our way through the dozens of remedies and preventatives there are for the common cold, it may help to clear the air, and our heads, if we consider what drug treatment your doctor will advise for a common cold if you call him in. Most doctors will advise: a couple of aspirin tablets to be taken as a start, with a hot drink (hot toddy, if

you wish); one aspirin tablet to be taken subsequently up to
three or four times a day to relieve any aches and pains; an
inhalant (probably Friars' Balsam) if your nose gets blocked
with thick secretion, and in the early stages a vasoconstrictor
spray or some drops, to be used not more than a few times and
only if you *must* get your nose really clear for a period. (There
are one or two sprays a doctor can prescribe that seem not to
have the disadvantages of the patent medicine sprays we discussed earlier). In a small minority of cases, where he is worried about those bacteria that may cause trouble after a virus
infection has started, he may prescribe an antibiotic, though the
risks that go with antibiotics are certainly not justified in the
vast majority of cases of the common cold.

Incidentally, there is some evidence that one day we shall
perhaps have a special kind of antibiotic that will act against
the common cold viruses; though not in this decade. Also, a
fairly effective vaccine against the common cold is at least on
the horizon: the trouble about making effective cold vaccines
has been the great variety of viruses involved, some of them
with a large family of relations, and some able to alter their
whole make-up from time to time; and the fact that the anti-
virus substances produced by the body in response to the cold
vaccine must be, not in the blood (as is the case with most infectious diseases), but in the nose and throat fluids. However,
there are signs that the various difficulties in the way of making
an effective vaccine may be overcome before too long.

12

Cough Sweets and
Cough Medicines

T H E C O M M O N or garden cough has as its object the expulsion from the chest or throat of unwanted material, or what the body thinks is unwanted material. This material is usually that white, glairy substance called mucus that we're all acquainted with; and it is produced by the throat or lungs as a result of irritation of one kind or another. Coughing is a very powerful and efficient mechanism: at the height of a cough, just when air is being forced most rapidly out of the throat, its speed through the throat is 760 mph.

However, that 760 mph blast is used not only when there is some mucus or other material to be got rid of (and free to move), but also when the body merely 'thinks' there is. If one has a *dry* inflammation of the throat or bronchial tubes, with some swelling of the lining membrane, one will very often cough to 'get rid' of non-existent mucus. What the body is really trying to get rid of is the inflamed membrane (which it mistakes for mucus), though, of course, it fortunately never succeeds. It can, however, make the inflammation of the membrane much worse with its repeated forceful coughing.

Doctors describe this type of cough as a dry or unproductive or useless cough; and one can also have such a cough when there is mucus present but it can't be brought up because it is dry and is clinging to the bronchial or throat membrane, or when the muscle of the bronchial tubes has gone into spasm, and so won't release the mucus. This occurs in asthma, and sometimes in bronchitis. The other kind of cough, the kind that does result in one's bringing up some mucus, is called a useful or productive cough. The mucus may, of course, contain material like dust particles, or be mixed with yellow pus (or even blood); the medical term for the complete product being sputum.

What is it that irritates the breathing passages so that they produce mucus and so cause a cough? A germ infection or virus infection is often present; a tumour can produce a cough; so can dust or fumes; and so can smoke. Often more than one cause is at work. In this country probably the commonest single cause of coughing is smoke: apart from the isolated cough brought on by a whiff of smoke, there is now no real doubt that long-continued cigarette smoking causes, not only lung cancer, but that common, slow-killing, coughing English disease, chronic bronchitis. It is aided and abetted by smog, which can sometimes 'go it alone'.

If you are a young person, and do not want your middle age and any old age you might be lucky enough to have – if you don't want them to be one long cough, don't start cigarette smoking, or, if you have started it, give it up. And if you're a middle-aged cigarette smoker, still give it up because something can be gained by doing so, even after years and years of smoking. (I haven't mentioned old cigarette smokers because, when one is old, the giving up of a habit is usually worse than any harm the habit can be causing; and in any case, for obvious reasons, there are few old people who smoke cigarettes.)

It is a sad irony that newspapers in this country carry advertisements both for cigarettes and for medicines to relieve the coughs that cigarettes cause. Government action – positive action, as well as just the forbidding of cigarette advertisements on television – is needed; but, of course, Governments of every political colour are conscious of how much money the tax on cigarettes brings in. Governments are conscious, too, of the many difficulties in the way of getting rid of our smoking chimneys. Difficulties, however, are made to be overcome, and it is a poor epitaph for any man, Government Minister or would-be non-smoker, that would read: 'He remained conscious of all the difficulties – until he ceased to be conscious of anything at all'.

Pending the smoke-free millennium, what can the ordinary person do about a cough? First, when should one go to a doctor with a cough, and when can one afford to treat oneself with a patent medicine? A cough should take you to your doctor if it lasts more than a week, or if it has come on without any obvious cause, or if there is much pain with it or a very high temperature or any sort of temperature lasting more than forty-eight hours, or if the sputum contains blood or yellow pus.

This still, of course, leaves quite a few mild, short-lived coughs that can be safely treated with homely cough remedies. So now what is in the patent medicines for coughs? And which should one choose for a particular kind of cough? First, one should distinguish between those cough remedies – mostly liquid, though some are in tablet form – that are meant to be swallowed more or less straight away, and those that are meant to be sucked, so that whatever is in them is swallowed only gradually. In general, the first kind is best for a chesty cough, and the second for a throaty cough. The liquid medicines have their own special types of ingredients, which are not usually found in the throat sweets; although the ingredients of throat sweets are mostly found in the liquid cough medicines also.

Throat sweets then – pastilles, lozenges, cough drops, etc. – are meant for throaty coughs, associated with a pharyngitis (throat inflammation), with the common cold, and so on. (Some of them, strictly speaking, are for the treatment of sore throats only and not of cough; but the two types of preparation are quite similar in composition and in effect, and they will, therefore, be treated together.) These preparations usually contain two or three types of ingredient. First is an antiseptic, intended to kill the germs that often cause this type of cough; and among these antiseptics are creosote, benzoin (or its tincture), thymol, cetyl pyridinium chloride, amylmetacresol, and chloroxylenol, the last three being more modern than the others.

Some of you, however, may remember what we said towards the end of Chapter 2 about antiseptics in general; and while certain of the antiseptics included in these throat sweets are ex-cellent purely as antiseptics – that is, if put with some germs in a test-tube – they can be much less effective inside the body. The throat, after all, has a number of warm nooks and crannies in which germs can safely lurk; and germs can lie 'doggo' in mucus or pus; and if an antiseptic ever did succeed in clearing the throat of them, there would be plenty more germs in the nose that would colonize the throat again in no time at all. If you suck antiseptic throat sweets all day long (and you might thereby make yourself sick), you will probably keep down the number of throat germs somewhat; but that's the best one can say about such sweets, at least as regards their antiseptic con-tent – though many of them do contain other substances as well. And one can say much the same about antiseptic gargles, which probably owe any value they have to the fact that the fluid in them helps to cleanse the throat.

The second group of substances commonly found in the various kinds of throat sweet are demulcents, or soothing sub-stances; which are soothing because they form a protective layer on the lining membrane of the throat. The commonly used demulcents are honey, liquorice (glycyrrhiza), and glycerin. They also help to produce a soothing flow of saliva, and they are aided in this by the sweetening agents in throat sweets (sucrose, liquid glucose), and also by the third group of ingredients, the essential oils and the miscellaneous sub-stances.

We have come across the essential oils before, of course – in the treatment of flatulence, and in treatments for the common cold. And some of the stronger of them also appear as counter-irritants in rheumatic rubs. 'What very versatile substances!' you may be saying. The fact is that, until we began thirty or forty years ago to obtain our modern, very powerful types of drug, essential oils were useful. Not because they would really cure anything, but because they were safe, and had a number of helpful little actions in the body, and above all because their taste and smell made them impressive to patients. Among the oils used in cough sweets are eucalyptus oil, peppermint oil (ol.

menth. pip.), aniseed oil (ol. anis.), cinnamon oil, lemon oil, ol. allii (from garlic), and clove oil (ol. caryoph.).

Apart from their taste and smell, they act as mild antiseptics in the throat and they stimulate the flow of saliva, as the demulcents do. In addition, it is said that, after they have been swallowed and taken into the bloodstream from the stomach, they are carried to the lungs and there stimulate the production of bronchial fluid, which might be soothing and help to carry away any germs; and also have a local antiseptic action in the bronchi, which, of course, might be very useful in the case of a chesty cough due to an infection. However, no doctor today takes *this* very seriously. (He uses antibiotics for a chest infection.) Indeed, no modern doctor takes essential oils very seriously at all. They're pleasant to take, and that's the chief thing about them.

Because they have a roughly similar action, one can classify with the essential oils a whole mass of miscellaneous substances often included in cough pastilles, lozenges, and so on. Among them are camphor, menthol, phenol, capsicum, chloroform, ether, and methyl salicylate. Some of them are included because they're antiseptic, some because they're mildly stimulating to the throat or nose, some because they're mild pain-relievers; and most of them do have an interesting taste or smell, and therefore probably stimulate the flow of saliva.

We keep coming back to this question of the flow of saliva. When one has a sore throat, saliva will help to wash away any undesirable débris (plus antiseptics, essential oils, and so on), and it will cover the inflamed throat membrane with a soothing liquid film. This is probably the chief benefit obtained from sucking throat sweets of any kind; and, of course, as the taste and smell of these sweets (due to their essential oils) makes one want to go on sucking them, the soothing, cleansing flow of saliva is kept up. Throat sweets, in other words, are pleasant, comforting, and harmless; but an ordinary sweet would usually do almost as much good, and would usually be cheaper.

The liquid cough medicines: most of them contain certain essential oils and/or one or two out of that group of miscellaneous substances we have just mentioned, plus sweetening agents. Some of them also contain demulcents, and one or two contain antiseptics. In addition, however, many of them contain extra substances, which really do act against cough, or have some other important action, once they're absorbed into the body.

What about those that *don't*? Those that contain just essential oils, and so on? What good can they possibly do? Well, they will all have a pleasant taste and smell, and those that are very thick and syrupy (the linctuses) will form a soothing coat over the throat membranes for a short time. Otherwise, it has to be admitted, there doesn't seem much point in putting into a liquid cough medicine, which one is going to swallow pretty quickly, substances that are mostly meant to act locally on the throat – in so far as such substances do have any worth-while action at all. Some of these cough medicines, for instance, contain antiseptics, and it's difficult to see what good *they* do when the medicines are quickly swallowed – none to the stomach certainly. It has been said that one should hold a cough linctus or medicine in one's mouth and throat for some time and so give the essential oils, etc., time to act on the lining membranes. However, few people seem to do this, and no one could keep a liquid medicine in his mouth and throat for anything like as long as he could keep on sucking a throat pastille.

The majority of these liquid cough remedies do also contain certain extra substances – to suppress cough, or to stimulate it, or to make one's chest feel easier. Some contain two such substances, some even contain three. First, then, those that suppress cough. What exactly is the nervous mechanism behind a cough? Coughing, although it can to some extent be controlled by an effort of will, is largely a reflex action: once there is some mucus or other material in the bronchi (bronchial tubes) to be got rid of, a message goes up the nerves of sensation to the spinal cord and to the cough centre in the brain, and then very quickly a message comes down the nerves going to the chest and throat muscles, and in no time at all one has coughed.

Cough suppressants must weaken or suppress this action

somewhere along the route taken by these messages; and usually they act on the cough centre in the brain. (The soothing substances found in many throat sweets, and the saliva itself, help to suppress cough, of course, by affecting the cough reflex at its start – by making the messages going from the throat lining up to the brain less frequent or less urgent.)

Among the cough suppressants used in patent medicine cough medicines are codeine and a substance called dextro-methorphan; but although the right amounts of substances such as these almost certainly can suppress many coughs some patent medicines do not contain an effective amount in a dose. Perhaps this isn't always a drawback because certain of these substances, as well as suppressing cough, have other actions that are most undesirable; and on the whole anyone who has a useless, unproductive cough and feels it needs something quite powerful to suppress it ought to go and see his doctor, and not simply take a patent medicine – at least he shouldn't continue taking one for more than a few days.

It is sometimes said that cough suppressants are also dangerous because, by stopping a person bringing up fluid from his chest, they might make him 'drown' in his own sputum. In fact, there is no evidence that they ever do this, or that they ever stop a cough that is really needed.

The second type of extra substance found in liquid cough medicines is a stimulant expectorant. Substances of this kind are irritant to the stomach, and this property enables them, by means of a reflex action, to increase the amount of fluid produced by the tiny glands in the bronchi. The person will then find it easier, so the story goes, to bring up his sputum, and in addition the fluid will form a soothing layer on the surface of the inflamed bronchi and so make coughing less frequent. Alas! it is a beautiful hypothesis, but it is doubtful whether – with most of these substances – anything of the kind ever happens, for the simple reason that the amounts of expectorants needed to produce this reflex effect would probably so irritate the stomach that the person taking them would also vomit. This isn't surprising if one remembers that coughing and vomiting are very similar actions – they're both methods of getting rid of unwanted material from the body.

However, whether or not they work, these stimulant expectorants have been used for many, many years, and do find their way into dozens of cough medicines, both the sort prescribed by doctors and the patent medicine sort. Among the stimulant expectorant substances found in the latter are ammonium acetate and chloride, antimony and potassium tartrate (another name for which is tartar emetic – 'emetic' meaning a substance to make one vomit), sodium benzoate, ipecacuanha, squill (scilla), tolu, Friars' Balsam (tinct. benzoin. co.), and creosote (made from wood tar). These last two substances, it has been said, are also absorbed and find their way via the blood stream to the bronchi, where they increase the flow of bronchial fluid and perhaps act as antiseptics. Readers may remember what was said about the similar, alleged property of essential oils.

The third and last kind of extra substance contained in liquid cough medicines (and in some chest tablets that are meant to be swallowed straight away) will ease one's chest by relaxing tight muscle in the bronchial tubes. These substances, which exert their effect after being absorbed from the stomach into the blood stream and being carried to the lungs, certainly do work. You will remember that one cause of a dry, unproductive cough can be that the bronchial tubes are tightly closed on the sputum the body is trying to cough up; so that these bronchodilators, as they're called, will ease one's cough (if it's of this kind) as well as one's chest – the bronchi relax, the sputum is coughed up, and the patient feels better. In addition they reduce the inflammatory swelling of the lining membrane of the bronchi. The names of some of these relaxing substances are: ephedrine, theophylline, theobromine, stramonium, and phenylephrine. However, as with the cough suppressants, people who feel they need cough medicines containing bronchodilators would probably be best advised to visit their doctors. The underlying condition, when the bronchial tubes are in spasm, is often chronic and it may be serious.

And lastly, just to make things a bit harder, a bronchodilator or a cough suppressant substance, or a stimulant expectorant is occasionally included in a cough *sweet* – that is, something meant to be sucked over a period.

The reader who has managed to thread his way through this jungle of cough medicine ingredients is probably, like the author, feeling rather confused; so let me console him by saying that we can't be half as confused as the manufacturers of some of these cough remedies. The bronchodilators they use certainly do 'work' and the cough suppressants and demulcents almost certainly do, but it is doubtful whether most of the stimulant expectorants really do anything of value (at least in the doses commonly used), and much the same can be said of the antiseptics, and the essential oils and miscellaneous ingredients. Indeed, it is probably to a great extent because of doubt as to whether the ingredients really work that most cough remedies contain so many of them. I say 'really' because a person in hospital will often believe and say that a cough medicine has relieved a cough when, in fact, a doctor or nurse will know from observation that he or she is coughing just as much as before.

For some unknown reason ten seems to be much the commonest number of ingredients found in a patent medicine cough remedy, though one or two contain eleven, and quite a number contain seven, eight, or nine. Some are doubtless included only for the sake of their taste or smell; but when a medicine of any kind contains more than three allegedly active ingredients (some doctors would say more than two), it is usually a safe bet that none of them is of much value, at any rate in the amounts included in the medicine. And sometimes, even when an ingredient of a cough medicine definitely possesses an action that is of value, it is included in amounts insufficient to exert this action. Such substances, of course, if present in amounts sufficient to produce a worth-while beneficial action will very often also have an undesirable action as well; and the manufacturer is aware of this, and plays safe.

Lastly – though this particular practice is one that is very common among doctors too – the patent medicine manufacturers often include in a single cough remedy two substances with apparently contradictory actions. For instance, a drug to suppress cough may be included alongside a drug to stimulate cough. Now, in fact, although it might seem to be the height of irrationality, this particular contradictory combination does seem to work quite well in practice – at least, so doctors find. Perhaps it is that the stimulant expectorant simply has no action at all, or else, if it has got an action, it produces an increase in bronchial fluid, which, after an initial clearing of the chest, actually soothes the bronchi and diminishes the amount of coughing – just as the cough suppressant will. In other words, the two have the same effect in the long run. Anyway, for whatever reason, the two do seem to harmonize, in much the same way as a powerful purge and a carminative.

Things become a little more difficult to swallow, however, when a bronchodilator ingredient is added to the other two. And they become almost impossible to swallow when eleven distinct substances are included in a single medicine. But then the manufacturer knows that many people are impressed by a medicine that contains a lot of ingredients, and he is never sure what kind of cough his medicine will be taken for; so he includes a little of everything and hopes to please everyone. This is traditional with cough medicines. It is also economical.

And now – what *should* one do if one has a cough? What would doctors recommend? Well, if it is the kind of cough that can properly be treated with home remedies, one should decide first whether it's a chesty cough or a throaty cough. (Any cough in or below the voice box is chesty, and any cough above it is throaty.) If it's throaty, then a cough sweet – of whatever colour and flavour you fancy – should help; although an ordinary kind of sweet will probably do almost as much good. A cough linctus, or a liquid cough medicine, will not do much good locally in the throat, but, if it contains a cough suppressant, it may have a beneficial effect after it's been swallowed down and absorbed from the stomach.

If you have a chesty cough, then steam inhalations will very often help; the steam making any dry, gummy mucus more

liquid and so easier to cough up. The addition of some Friars'
Balsam to the steaming water will provide a comforting, antiseptic smell, and the balsam *may* even stimulate the bronchi to
produce some fluid or else act as an antiseptic (in much the
same way as the essential oils in cough pastilles provide a local
treatment to the lining membrane of the throat). Any of the
inhalants we discussed in the last chapter could be used instead
of Friars' Balsam.

What else would a doctor recommend? Just possibly a cough
suppressant medicine for a dry cough. And apart from keeping
in a warm and reasonably moist atmosphere, that's all. In a
nutshell, sweets for the throat, steam and Friars' Balsam for
the chest. Minor coughs, you see, will clear up in a matter of
days, irrespective of what treatment they get, although the
measures suggested will at least make the waiting period somewhat easier. Of course, if you *want* to take a cough medicine
that may not do you much good but does at least taste pleasant
and interesting, there'll be no harm in taking it – so long as you
don't, because you're taking it, put off going to your doctor
when you know you should.

If you have a *chronic* cough, your doctor will probably tell
you that a simple hot drink (it doesn't much matter what) will
help you bring up the phlegm (or sputum), especially first thing
in the morning.

We said earlier that gargles are not of any great value when
one has a cough. The same can be said of throat sprays, which
in any case are not especially popular. The only kind of remedy
we still have not considered is the sort that's meant to be
rubbed on the chest or throat. As we mentioned in the last
chapter, the fumes from such a remedy act as an inhalation;
but in addition, it is said that, owing to the irritant action of
the ingredients of these rubs, they reflexly improve the circulation of the deeper tissues – in particular, of the lungs if they're
applied to the chest. It's difficult to be sure of whether this
would do any good, if it happened. Conceivably it might. However, it's even more difficult to be sure of whether it does, in
fact, happen: though, as we mentioned when dealing with

rheumatic balms, the smell of these rubs may so fill a person's mind that there's no room for anything else – thoughts of pain or discomfort, for instance.

The last thing to be said in this chapter is that, if anyone knows why we don't all drown when we have a bad cold, he might make his knowledge public. One can have a streaming cold (often with a cough), which uses up perhaps a dozen handkerchiefs a day; one can have a nose that's almost running water; and yet when one goes to bed and sleeps this tap is somehow turned off. If it wasn't turned off, if the secretion into the nose continued at the same rate as when we're awake, then more than enough fluid would be produced in eight hours of sleep to drown one. As we all know, very little fluid is produced, in fact. We wake up with a dry, crusted nose – and ten minutes later, when we're on our feet, we're sneezing, and pouring out great volumes of fluid again. Why? Medical science doesn't yet know; but it's a small personal hunch that, if we did know why, we might well be on the way to discovering the best cold remedy of all.

13

Vitamins

ONE WOULD never believe that four small letters of the alphabet could create a medium-sized industry, but that is what happened in the case of vitamins. Not the four letters that stand for the four common vitamins – A, B, C, and D, but the letters V-I-T-A that start the word 'Vitamins'. They also start the word 'vitality', and so for years millions of people have felt that vitamins mean vitality, that one only has to take them regularly and one will be full of energy, optimism, sparkle, gaiety, and *joie de vivre*. In fact, most of the vitamins that are hopefully taken by people in this country who are wanting to have all those wonderful qualities are sooner or later thrown out of the body without making the least difference to it. Most people in this country, you see, are not short of vitamins at all.

It is true that, if one *is* really short of vitamins – if, that is, one has an illness clearly due to lack of vitamins – one will usually be short of energy, optimism, etc., as well; but that will be the least of your worries. And there are plenty of other conditions that cause a lack of vitality, most of them very much commoner, at least in this country, than a lack of vitamins. A neurosis, for instance, or a middle-aged depression, or an anaemia, or almost any chronic smouldering illness – all these produce a lack of vitality. And taking vitamins if one is suffering from such a condition will not have the slightest beneficial effect. If vitamins had been called, let us say, 'minifactors' in the very first place, then they would probably not have become nearly so popular as they are.

All this is not to deny that extra vitamins are of some value to a minority of people in this country, and, as part of a proper diet, would be of value to millions of malnourished (i.e. starving) people in countries overseas. So let us look at them a little more closely, and scientifically. Vitamins are definite chemical compounds that the body needs to obtain from food in small quantities if it is to function properly. They are quite distinct from the carbohydrates, fats, and proteins that we also get from our food, and are also distinct from the minerals like iron and calcium. Indeed, vitamins are to the rest of one's diet roughly what salt is to a stew or yeast is to bread. As we all know, vitamins are named after the letters of the alphabet, although they also have chemical names (like ascorbic acid or aneurine), most of which are used only by doctors and pharmacists – and even by them only on solemn occasions.

The patent medicine type of vitamin preparation (the kind you buy at a pharmacy counter) is nearly always an oily liquid or a fruity one or else a tablet or capsule. The oily liquids consist of a fish liver oil, like cod or halibut liver oils, though sometimes they have 'tonic' substances added; and they supply vitamins A and D. The fruity liquids consist of orange juice, or blackcurrant or rose hip syrup; and they supply vitamin C mainly. And lastly, the tablets or capsules usually contain a number of vitamins, often with minerals as well; though few of them contain only a single vitamin, or perhaps two major vitamins – as, for example, capsules containing cod liver oil.

And now let us look at the vitamins one by one. They can be divided into two groups: first, those that are soluble in fats – vitamins A, D, E, and K; second, those that are soluble in water – the B vitamins, and vitamin C.

The first of them, vitamin A, is found in milk, butter, cheese, liver, and egg yolk – and perhaps you've noticed that all these foods contain some fat, in which the vitamin A is dissolved. It is also found in margarines and infant foods, because vitamins A and D are added to these. Much the commonest rich sources of vitamin A (and of vitamin D) that one can buy are cod and halibut liver oils, but there is no vitamin A (or any other vitamin) in any of the ordinary vegetable oils, like olive oil, sunflower seed oil, maize oil, cottonseed oil, and groundnut oil, which are used in cooking.

There is, however, one vegetable oil that can supply vitamin A, and that is the red palm oil of West Africa, which is extensively used there for cooking purposes. It can *supply* vitamin A, although it does not actually contain any of the vitamin: it contains instead a substance called carotene, which is a provitamin. That means the body can change it into vitamin A, so that for all practical purposes any foods rich in carotene are rich in vitamin A. Carotene is the substance in carrots that gives them their colour; and it is present also in tomatoes, apricots, and the dark green leaves of vegetables. It also gives their yellow colour to butter and egg yolk; and to those few people who eat enormous amounts of carotene-containing foods – for example, the American lady whose doctor a few years ago was puzzled by her colour until he found out she was drinking three and a half pints of tomato juice every single day.

Disease due to a lack of vitamin A is serious, but it is practically never seen in this country. It occurs not uncommonly in parts of Asia, and among other things gives rise to night blindness, to a thickening of the horny layer of the skin round the mouths of the skin's sweat and oil glands, and to a similar change in certain lining membranes of the body, including those of the bronchial tubes. Because a severe lack of vitamin A over a long period may have this effect, it has been argued that vitamin A might be of value to people whose night vision is poor, or to people with colds (which, of course, affect some of the body's lining membranes), or to people with certain skin disorders – acne, for instance.

This is a type of false reasoning that has been applied time and again to the vitamins: because a gross lack of a vitamin produces a certain bodily change, then whenever a change of that kind occurs, or an illness that *might* be produced by such a change, it must be treated with the vitamin, preferably in huge doses. So the argument goes. It is a false argument, because the change or illness may well have some other cause than a vitamin lack; and in practice they nearly always do

have. For instance, although the common cold certainly does
affect the lining membranes of the breathing passages, it is
not caused by any change in them but by a virus infection, and
it affects people who are getting plenty of vitamin A in their
food. And again, night blindness in this country is commonly
due to fatigue, or to a type of inflammation of the retina of the
eye, and very, very rarely to a lack of vitamin A. What's more,
in practice no convincing evidence has been produced that,
in the absence of a vitamin A deficiency, large doses of the
vitamin have any effect at all on either of these two conditions
– or on acne for that matter.

A story from the 1939–45 war shows how wrong, but how
widely believed, some of these vitamin myths may be. A
rumour was going about at one stage that R A F pilots had
started to eat lots of carrots for the sake of the carotene in
them, and that the vitamin A this had given them had enormously improved their night vision. They now had eyes like
lynxes, it was said: that was why they were suddenly shooting
down dozens of German planes at night over this country.
Perhaps the Germans believed it. Certainly a lot of Britishers
did. However, the truth of the matter was that radar had just
been introduced, and we wanted to keep the fact of its existence secret for as long as possible. Some of the peace-time
myths about vitamins are just as far from the truth as that
rumour, and with much less justification. And many of them
are kept alive by the advertisements of the patent medicine
manufacturers.

An excess of vitamin A is occasionally given by accident,
usually by mothers who believe their children can't have too
much of a good thing. In fact, of course, practically all things
are bad if taken to excess, and vitamin A is no exception. These
mothers will give a very concentrated liquid preparation of
vitamin A in spoonful doses when the proper dose for a child
is just a few drops – for instance, halibut liver oil (a very concentrated source of vitamins A and D) in the teaspoonful doses
she would quite rightly use for cod liver oil (which is a much
less concentrated source). Another, and less common way to

make sure you will suffer from vitamin A poisoning is to eat some polar bear's liver for lunch. It is an extremely rich source of vitamin A, and the Eskimos have learnt from experience never to touch it.

An excess of vitamin A causes loss of appetite, vomiting, headache, and dryness of the skin: it is a serious condition, particularly in infants. And the best way to prevent it is to take any preparation containing vitamin A only in the doses given on the label – if, that is, you must take it at all. But please don't think, if your baby vomits, that he's suffering from vitamin A poisoning: it's still a pretty uncommon condition, and your baby will be in no danger at all of getting it so long as you stick to the doses of halibut or cod liver oil recommended by your doctor or at your clinic, or on the bottle label.

Two final points about vitamin A. Fish liver oils do lose some of the vitamin they contain if they're left exposed to sunlight for a long time in a glass bottle. Second, cod liver oil contains what are called unsaturated fatty acids, which some doctors believe may help to prevent the coronary heart disease that middle-aged men often have. Certainly cod liver oil will lower the level of cholesterol in the blood, and most doctors would agree that a high level is undesirable. However, before he starts swigging a tablespoonful or two of cod liver oil every day, any worried middle-aged businessman should consult his doctor, and be guided by what *he* says.

Vitamin D is the second of the fat-soluble vitamins, and the only other very important one. A marked lack of vitamin D causes rickets, the well-known disease of bones that was once very common indeed among young children in this country, and that still occurs here now and again. Until about forty years ago there was a lot of medical argument as to whether rickets was due to some deficiency in the diet, or to a lack of sunshine (for it commonly affected poor children who were inadequately fed but who also lived in dark cities). We know nowadays that both theories were right. We know that vitamin D is not only present in certain foods, but is actually formed in the skin when sunlight plays upon it; and that the body's vitamin D comes from *both* sources. A deficiency in food or in sunlight (or in both) can therefore produce rickets.

As well as there being more than one source for the body's vitamin D, there is more than one kind of the vitamin. The vitamin D we get from foods, and that is formed in our skin, is called vitamin D_3; but a very similar substance, that will also prevent or cure rickets, can be produced artificially. It is called vitamin D_2, or calciferol. In practice either sort of vitamin D is probably quite satisfactory for man.

Vitamin D is found in milk, butter, egg yolk, liver, and other animal foods containing fat; and it is also added to margarine and some infant foods. And cod liver and halibut liver oils, and fatty fish, contain a lot of it. What vitamin D does is to control the absorption by the body of the calcium present in foodstuffs, and also the 'laying down' of this calcium in the bones. When there is a lack of vitamin D, food calcium passes right through the body, and because of the body's lack of it the bones become soft. The ends of the limb bones get bigger and the shafts of the leg bones bend under the body weight, producing bow legs or knock knees (if the child has started to walk). Bosses (knobbly lumps) appear on the skull, and a peculiar beading on the ribs. And a baby with rickets is pale, flabby, irritable, and late in walking. Most of the few babies who suffer from rickets in this country today are the children of coloured immigrants; and the chief cause of their condition is that their skins apparently do not receive enough sunlight in this country to produce worth-while amounts of vitamin D; though a lack of cod or halibut liver oil, and of foods fortified with vitamin D, may also be important.

Very large doses of vitamin D have been used in the treatment of various skin conditions, but in only one – a condition called lupus vulgaris – was it ever proved to be of value, and even for that condition it has now been replaced by other drugs. Vitamin D can be taken to dangerous excess, either by being deliberately consumed in very large doses (in the hope of improving a skin condition, for example), or 'accidentally' in the same way as an excess of vitamin A can be taken. Big doses produce a state of vitamin D poisoning, with vomiting, loss of appetite, constipation, weakness, and drowsiness.

There is one form of this vitamin D poisoning that occurred fairly often in infants a few years ago. Infants receive the vitamin not only from cod liver oil or halibut liver oil, but from infant foods, dried milk, and even from margarine, to all of which vitamin D is deliberately added by the manufacturers on expert medical advice. It was estimated a few years ago that, as a result, quite a few infants were receiving as much as five times the amount of vitamin D they really needed. Experts, you see, *can* sometimes go astray. The basic cause of the illness these infants had – so some doctors thought – was not the excess of vitamin D but the fact that they were unduly sensitive to its action. But, whatever the exact cause, the amount of vitamin D being added to infant foods, etc., was dropped a few years ago, and since then (though not immediately) the number of cases of this disease of young children has also dropped.

It is in part because of this that many doctors have given up the habit – a very good one twenty or thirty years ago – of automatically advising vitamin supplements for all infants and young children, as well as for all nursing and expectant mothers. Our diets today are usually more than adequate, and expectant mothers and probably nursing mothers do not need any vitamin supplements *if* they are taking a good mixed diet. As for children, if they are taking milks and cereals fortified with vitamin D they probably do not need any extra vitamin D from cod liver oil or similar supplement; though a breast-fed child, or one fed cow's milk only, should take such a supplement particularly during the winter months. One should be guided in all this by the advice of one's doctor or clinic; and one should always stick to the dosage of the oil recommended on the bottle label. In that way the baby won't be given a dangerous amount of vitamin D – or of vitamin A, which is nearly always found in the same supplements as vitamin D.

There are two other fat-soluble vitamins – E and K. Although a great deal of work has been done with vitamin E (and even more in producing learned papers about it), no one has ever shown that a lack of it causes any disease in man, or that giving extra vitamin E has any beneficial effect at all. Also, large doses appear not to do any harm. In other words, as far as we can tell, no one at all needs any extra vitamin E, though you won't hurt anything but your pocket if you *do* take a big dose of it every day.

Vitamin K is involved in the clotting of the blood, and a shortage of it produces a 'bleeding' illness. However, such a shortage, in adults at any rate, is always itself caused by some other serious disease, for which the attention of a doctor will have been needed anyway. In other words, a lack of vitamin K is not something the reasonably healthy man in the street need bother his head about; and in fact, you're very unlikely to find vitamin K in any patent medicine vitamin product.

And now we come to the B vitamins, and vitamin C, which are the water-soluble vitamins. There is not just one B vitamin, but ten or eleven, though some of them, like pantothenic acid, biotin, and inositol, are of no practical importance to man. A good food source of one B vitamin is usually, though not invariably, a good source of others; and yeast and liver are particularly rich in the B complex – as the whole collection of B vitamins is sometimes called. Many other common foods contain one or more members of the complex; and naturally, when a person is short of one B vitamin, he is usually short of some of the others as well. However, disease due to a lack of B vitamins is uncommon in this country, though it can occur – in alcoholics (who are not getting enough good food into themselves), in people with some internal condition that prevents them absorbing their food properly, and in people with such strange beliefs about foods, so strongly held, that they do not give themselves a proper diet.

Some of these people, of course, will be receiving medical treatment anyway, and so their doctors will be watching their intake of B vitamins. And those who aren't will nearly always be uninterested in taking extra vitamins or be unwilling to. In other words, there is no case at all for advising any group of people in this country to take extra B vitamins in patent medicine form in order to prevent a deficiency.

That being said, let us look very quickly at the more important of the B vitamins. A lack of vitamin B_1 (or aneurine or thiamine, as it is called) leads to beri-beri, a serious condition, most often seen in the Far East, and due to eating a lot of over-refined carbohydrate food and little else. For instance, a diet consisting largely of polished rice (that is, rice from which the vitamin-containing husk has been removed) will produce beri-beri. Its importance here is that among its early symptoms are irritability, forgetfulness, and depression – all of them symptoms that occur in certain common neurotic illnesses. Because such symptoms, when due to beri-beri, can be cured by giving vitamin B_1, people have thought that vitamin B_1 should always be given whenever such symptoms occurred (in neurosis, for example); which, of course, is nonsense. Other symptoms in beri-beri are weakness and pains and numbness of the legs, due to the lack of vitamin B_1 affecting the patient's nervous system; and, therefore, very often, when a person has *these* symptoms, he gets vitamin B_1 too, though the symptoms nearly always have some cause very much commoner than any lack of B_1.

Riboflavine, or vitamin B_2, is not of great importance. A lack of it causes a rash, cracking of the skin at the corners of the mouth, and greasiness of the skin. Vitamin B_6, or pyridoxine, is also unimportant, an illness due to lack of it being extremely uncommon and usually caused by the taking of a particular drug. Like most vitamins, however, pyridoxine has been used hopefully in the treatment of a number of conditions: it is, in fact, of value in 'radiation sickness'; and *may* be of value in pregnancy vomiting. Two B vitamins that *are* very important are vitamin B_{12}, used in the treatment of pernicious anaemia, and folic acid, used in the treatment of some other kinds of anaemia, especially in pregnancy. A lack of B_{12}, we now realize, is present in certain mental illnesses and of folic acid in some old people. However, although these substances are most im-

portant, they are not found in patent medicine vitamin preparations.

Perhaps the most interesting of the common-or-garden B
vitamins is the one we've left till last – nicotinic acid. It has
nothing whatever to do with nicotine, although so many lay
people in the USA used to think it had that the authorities
there gave it the new name of niacin. A lack of nicotinic acid
produces the condition of pellagra, a disease in which there is
loss of appetite and weakness, a skin rash, mental changes, and
diarrhoea. Pellagra is still seen in various parts of the world,
and not so many years ago used to be seen in mental hospitals
in this country. One curious fact about pellagra is that it is
most commonly seen in areas where maize figures largely in the
diet (as in certain parts of the United States); and doctors now
believe this is, to a great extent, because maize is lacking in a
substance with the long name of tryptophane, out of which the
body can make nicotinic acid for itself.

Nicotinic acid is an interesting vitamin because, apart from
its value in pellagra (which is still fairly common, though *not*
in this country), it has been used for the treatment of a number
of conditions other than those due to vitamin lack, and with
more justification than there is for the widespread use of most
other vitamins. Nicotinic acid can help to relieve certain headaches, for instance; probably because it has the power of opening up small blood vessels. For the same reason it is used for
the treatment of chilblains. It has been claimed to give good
results in some cases of arthritis; and in big doses it will lower
a high blood cholesterol level. While the value of these uses is
not really established, it can at least be said for nicotinic acid
that in big doses it is not a poison, unlike vitamins A and D,
and it may even do some good. Incidentally, big doses of other
B vitamins do little harm – though most of them won't do any
good in big doses, unless you're truly short of them.

Lastly we have vitamin C, the vitamin that comes in fresh
fruits and vegetables. Blackcurrants are a rich source, and so
are rose hips, and citrus fruits – oranges, lemons, limes, grape-
fruit. British sailors became known as 'Limeys' because they

were given lime juice regularly to prevent scurvy, the disease caused by a lack of vitamin C. In fact, although vitamin C was unknown at the time, lime juice does not contain as much of the vitamin as lemon juice, and it did not prevent scurvy altogether. Vitamin C is easily destroyed, especially by heat; and alas! some over-conscientious mothers have religiously boiled their babies' orange juice every day – in order to sterilize it – thus ensuring that all its vitamin C was destroyed and that their babies got scurvy. Because vitamin C is easily destroyed in this way, fruit and vegetables are a better source of the vitamin when raw than when cooked – as well as often being much pleasanter to eat. In order to preserve their vitamin C, vegetables that have to be cooked should be boiled in the minimum of water for the least time necessary to make them appetizing and digestible. The kind of cabbage that has been boiled for three-quarters of an hour in two pints of water with bicarbonate of soda added – that kind of cabbage contains no vitamin C worth mentioning, as well as being, in the eyes of any good cook, the ruin of a most noble vegetable.

Scurvy is still sometimes seen in this country – in artificially fed babies who are given no fruit juice or fruit syrup, and in old people who live on a diet of tea, bread and margarine, and fish and chips. The patient with scurvy complains of weakness, and of bone pains; and he shows bruising of the skin and bleeding into it, swelling and bleeding of the gums, and loosening of the teeth. Wounds will not heal properly, and the scars of old wounds sometimes break down. So long as they are taking a full, mixed diet, nursing and expectant mothers and toddlers do not actually *need* a vitamin C supplement; though infants, particularly bottle-fed infants, probably do need one – to prevent scurvy. And so long as it is administered properly, a fruit juice vitamin C supplement, as well as being pleasant, will certainly not do the least harm to *any* of these groups.

However, one should never put a sugar-sweetened fruit juice product – or anything else that's sugary – in a baby's dummy, or in a miniature feeding bottle that is then left in the baby's cot for him to suck as he pleases: the sugar, helped by the

acid in the case of a fruit product, will cause the baby's teeth
to decay very badly. Syrupy fruit juice products should be
well diluted with water, and should then be fed to the baby by
the mother like an ordinary feed. There is now at least one
vitamin C supplement that is not sweetened with sugar, and
this would certainly seem preferable for babies and young
children.

Old people will get plenty of vitamin C if they take fresh
fruit or vegetable twice a day; but if there is any difficulty
about this, then they too should be encouraged to take one of
the fruit juice products, though these are certainly expensive
for some old people. Vitamin C is also available, more cheaply,
as a tablet and is then every bit as good as vitamin C from fruit.

Vitamin C in very big doses has been recommended for the
treatment of the common cold and similar conditions; and
smaller doses taken every day have been recommended to prevent one catching colds. There is some evidence that vitamin C
is of value when taken in this way, but it is not at all conclusive;
and on the whole the best one can say is that, if big doses of
vitamin C are taken, at least they will not do any harm.

This brings us back to what we wrote at the start of this
chapter, and it will bear repetition: the great majority of
people in this country are not short of any vitamin, and therefore there is no need at all for them to take any extra vitamins
in patent medicine or any other form. Those people who are
short of vitamins or who might become short (expectant and
nursing mothers, babies, old people, those who live alone,
patients on special diets, and people who eat strange diets, or
who have some disease preventing proper absorption of foods,
or who have had certain kinds of operation, or whose appetite
is poor over a long period) – most of these people should be
under the care of a doctor, and most of them will be; and he
will recommend any vitamins that may be needed.

Old people, especially if poor and living alone, and people
who eat strange diets may be exceptions: often they are unknown to any doctor, and alas! many of them will not take
good advice about what they should eat – from a doctor or

anyone else. It is nevertheless the duty of all of us to keep an eye on the food such people are getting, particularly old people; and to try to induce them to eat a healthy diet, or else to visit a doctor. Doing good by stealth is probably the best way. However, most of us can forget about vitamins otherwise. Eat a diet that includes a good helping of almost every kind of food every day, and your vitamins will look after themselves.

Minerals are often included in patent medicine vitamin preparations. Nobody in this country is short of manganese, one of the minerals included; very few are now short of iodine, which is another. Quite a number of people are short of iron, and even more *could* be short of calcium. However, people who are short of iron have an anaemia, which should be treated by a doctor and not by means of a patent medicine. In other words, if you feel exhausted, and are breathless or have palpitations – all possible symptoms of an anaemia – then go straight to your doctor.

The people who *could* be short of calcium are expectant and nursing mothers, and babies and young children. However, with the provision of cheap milk, and with the much better knowledge that most mothers now have of what they and their children should and should not eat, lack of calcium is, in fact, very uncommon. In other words, just as with vitamins, so long as we are having a reasonable diet, most of us needn't bother our heads about the minerals we're perhaps not getting. We're getting them all right. Indeed, the only mineral the worriers are likely to find themselves short of is silver.

14

Tonics

THE MONETARY value of tonics used in this country is very considerable: over £3 million a year is spent on patent medicine tonics alone. But the value of tonics to those who take them – the true medical value – is almost nil. Why is this? People take tonics because they are feeling tired, exhausted, unable to concentrate, 'run down', irritable, depressed, 'out-of-sorts', and so on. In other words, they take them for one or more of the items in a very mixed bag of vague symptoms.

Such symptoms are, however, very real to those who have them; and the conditions that can give rise to them are equally real. These symptoms (or some of them) can be due to an anaemia, for instance, or to a nervous (neurotic) illness, or a depression, or the early stages of almost any serious physical disease. They can occur in convalescence from illness, particularly influenza. And they can be due to worry, or unhappiness in love or at work, or lack of sleep or of food over a period.

Two things about tonics should now be obvious. First, that there are a great many widely different causes for people feeling run down, and therefore there cannot possibly be any *single* tonic medicine suitable for all of them. Second, that, when a person is run down, it will very often need a doctor to find out just what the underlying cause is, and to prescribe the proper treatment. This is particularly necessary if, as often obtains, the cause is a serious one. Now and again it is possible for a lay person to say with confidence that he (or some friend or relative) is run down because of some obvious upset in his personal life – too much work, perhaps; or a chronic disagreement with his wife. But in that case the first thing to do is to try and smooth out the disagreement or reduce the amount of work; and the second thing might be to have a holiday with plenty of good food and exercise. A bottle of medicine will do no good in such circumstances.

Certainly, when a doctor has found out just why some patient is feeling run down, *he* will often prescribe a bottle of medicine or some tablets, but his prescription will be suited to the individual patient. If the cause is an anaemia due to lack of iron, which in turn will often be due to chronic bleeding (from piles, for instance), the doctor will want to treat the piles, and he will also prescribe some iron in liquid or tablet form. If the cause is a depressive illness, which is common in middle-age, he may prescribe a modern anti-depressant drug. If the cause is some difficulty at home or at work, he will try and smooth it out, and perhaps give the patient a sedative drug for a month or so – until the patient has achieved the much better sedative of contentment at his home or his work.

There is, in fact, almost no end to the number of separate drugs a doctor may prescribe for different patients who are 'run down'. But those patients, if left to treat themselves, might well choose exactly the same popular patent medicine tonic in every case; and even if, in search of the 'right' tonic, they were to look along the tonic shelf in a chemist's shop, they wouldn't, in fact, see much real variety – dozens of labels certainly, but the actual contents of the bottles would justify one in saying there were only five separate kinds of patent medicine tonic.

The biggest single group is that of the vitamins, and we considered these in the last chapter. The other four groups are: those containing foods of one kind or another, those containing iron, those that contain yeast, and those that contain a nerve 'food' or a stimulant for the nervous system. There is a good deal of overlap of all the groups, but we shall now consider the value of each of these last four groups separately – on the assumption that it is possible for a lay person to know just why someone is feeling run down, and which kind of tonic might do him good, although, in fact, this cannot usually be done by anybody but a doctor.

First, then, the foods. These contain one or more of the following: casein (the protein in our everyday milk and cheese), bone marrow, egg, corn oil, malt, and so on (plus vitamins and/or hypophosphites and/or iron and other minerals). One's first reaction to the idea of buying one of these foods at a chemist's for a run-down person is to ask why one shouldn't buy some straightforward foods instead – at a grocer's or a butcher's or greengrocer's. Perhaps more expensive foods than usual (to tempt the appetite), but still foods, clearly recognizable as such. Any good housewife can, with the right ingredients and a little imagination, produce a meal that will tempt a jaded appetite much more than any tonic food to be got out of a tin or bottle.

If the person concerned won't eat even a meal of that kind, if he won't take anything at all by mouth or will take fluids only, then perhaps he or his stomach knows best. Perhaps his stomach is upset and needs a rest, or perhaps he is starting a feverish illness. If so, he is best left without any nourishment, apart from fluids possibly. And if his loss of appetite should last more than a day or so, he had better be seen by a doctor: a loss or diminution of appetite lasting for days or weeks *may* be a sign of serious illness. Such an illness, however, can quite often be cured if it is spotted early enough by a doctor. And by the way, even sillier than to attempt to treat a loss of appetite with one of the tonic foods is to treat a loss of weight with one of them: any loss of weight not due to a reducing diet should take you to your doctor straight away.

Some people imagine that these tonic foods have some very special quality not present in an ordinary meal. The only extra they do, in fact, have is their added hypophosphites, iron, etc., and we shall consider these in a moment. Their food ingredients are exactly the same as the basic ingredients of ordinary foods, and are often less tempting; and most important, they'll do you no more good than the ingredients of an ordinary three-meals-a-day diet.

Group 2 comprises the products containing iron. The iron is in the form of a salt such as ferrous sulphate or ferrous phosphate, and very often these products also contain some of the B vitamins or else yeast, which is a good source of B vitamins. Anaemia (that is, a poor quality of the blood) can be due to a shortage of body iron, and this kind of anaemia is quite common in this country, especially among women whose monthly 'loss' takes iron out of their bodies. We get iron chiefly from red meat and green vegetables, and a shortage of it in the body may be caused by a person's having eaten very little of the iron-rich foodstuffs over a long period, or by a chronic blood loss which has been taking iron out of the body faster than the best diet in the world can put it in – and often, in fact, the very people who are losing blood are not receiving even an average diet.

An anaemia can cause all kinds of symptoms, including a 'run-down' feeling; and when the anaemia is due to iron lack, these symptoms will vanish after a few weeks of treatment with an iron medicine. (Iron is useless in other, less common kinds of anaemia.) However, the basic cause of the anaemia, particularly if it is producing a loss of blood, must first be discovered and put right, and only a doctor can do this. (The cause *may* be serious, and the loss of blood may be a 'hidden' one.)

In addition, to cure an anaemia due to iron lack, iron must be given in quite large amounts, larger, in fact, than the amounts present in some of these patent medicine iron tonics. On the whole, therefore – quite apart from the fact that it is very difficult for a lay person to be certain that an anaemia is present, let alone an iron-deficiency anaemia – the use of these iron tonics cannot be recommended. And to use them blindly, because someone is exhausted or irritable or off his food, cannot be too strongly condemned. It may give an unreal and dangerous sense of security.

As well as the B vitamins or yeast that most of these iron tonics contain, some of them contain vitamin C. Occasionally vitamin C is of value in an iron-deficiency anaemia. But B vitamins and yeast are never necessary – they do no harm, but

they won't do any good either. Sometimes they also contain
manganese or copper, which make no difference at all to their
value; or caffeine, which we shall deal with later in this chapter; or an aperient. It used to be common practice, even with
doctors, to advise an aperient with an iron-containing medicine,
presumably on the ground that, if you needed toning up, you
also needed cleaning out. We now realize there is no good
reason for the combination. In any case, even though iron and
an unnecessary aperient still appear in the products of one or
two patent medicine manufacturers, they often don't put in
enough aperient for it to have any laxative action at all.

That mention of yeast just now brings us to Group 3 of the
tonic preparations – those that contain yeast, sometimes with
an analgesic (or pain-relieving) drug. Why should yeast be
thought of as a tonic? Perhaps because many years ago people
felt that, if it made bread rise, it would make them rise too.
And then, as we mentioned in the last chapter, yeast is a good
source of B vitamins, a severe shortage of which can certainly
lead to disease of the nerves – a true, physical disease, that is.
But many people who are run down are described as 'nervy'.
Therefore – so the argument goes – yeast should be of value to
them. One can spot various weak links in this case (which we
encountered first in Chapter 13). For a start, a shortage of B
vitamins is practically never seen in this country. And then
actual physical disease of the nerves is quite different from the
'nervous' disease that many run-down people have: theirs is a
disease of the mind, a neurosis. And lastly, nobody has ever
shown that giving yeast to run-down people will, in fact, improve all of them, or even a certain proportion of them. Yeast
won't do anyone much harm, but it won't do any good to most
people either. The place for it is in bread.

Just before we leave yeast – it is difficult to think of any
sensible reason for combining yeast with a pain-relieving drug,
although this is done in some patent medicine tonics. Even if
yeast was of value, it would need to be taken for days or weeks
before the B vitamins in it had any real effect. But pain-relieving drugs act in a matter of minutes, or, at worst, in an hour

or so. In other words, apart from the fact that analgesics and yeast are quite different substances, suitable for quite different kinds of complaint, they cannot possibly act 'together'. So why combine them? It's like serving steak and ice cream on the same plate. And finally, another name for yeast, sometimes used on labels, is Cerevis Ferment. Sicc., but what you get inside is still yeast.

The fourth and last kind of patent medicine contains either a stimulant to the nervous system or a special nerve 'food' for it. The stimulant is nearly always caffeine, the substance in tea and coffee that provides the 'lift' one gets from these two drinks. If a person is tired through having overworked for a day or two, caffeine may be of help, at least for a few hours; but it would be quite the wrong treatment for anyone who was truly run down. In such a person one should seek for the cause of the condition, not use a drug to 'whip' him into activity for a short time. And if one is simply tired, one can get a 'lift' more pleasantly from a cup of tea or coffee (or two cups) than from a caffeine tablet. The tablet might, of course, be convenient if one was feeling tired on the top of Mont Blanc or in the middle of the Brazilian jungle. But – are you?

And what about the special nerve 'foods', the alternative ingredient in this fourth group of tonics? These are just about the biggest bit of nonsense in the whole tonic field. The biggest selling too. Phosphorus is present in most parts of one's body. In particular, it is present in one's brain and one's nerves. Some of the phosphorus in this nervous tissue is present as glycerophosphates. Therefore, glycerophosphates must be good for the nerves. This is the 'evidence', the total argument, underlying the use of glycerophosphates and some substances called hypophosphites as tonics.

Let us look at one or two extra awkward facts. As far as doctors are concerned, no one has ever been shown to be ill as a result of shortage of these substances (glycerophosphates, or hypophosphites) in his body. Indeed, such a shortage is unknown. Also, when taken by mouth, glycerophosphates are broken down in one's digestive system: in other words, they cannot even reach one's nerve tissue. And when hypophosphites are taken, they are thrown out by the body unchanged: in other words, *they* don't get to the nerve tissue either. Finally, it has never been shown that giving glycerophosphates or hypophosphites has done any good to anybody. It is true that hypophosphites have been used in the treatment of tuberculosis, but not since 1855; and anyway, nobody showed, even then, that they had the least beneficial effect; and what has tuberculosis to do with nerves?

Despite all this, glycerophosphates and hypophosphites continue to appear in tonics, in some that are prescribed, as well as in the patent medicine sort. They are added to those foods that formed Group 1 in our classification of tonics (vitamins aside); they are mixed with cod liver oil, glycerin, and liquid paraffin to give another kind of tonic; they have bitters added to them to give another; and they are even mixed into tonic wines. And after all that, the best one can say about them is that they're harmless to the body, if not to the purse.

The bitters we mentioned just now were considered in some detail in Chapter 7, but here are a few words about tonic wines. Strictly speaking, they are not patent medicine, but they *are* sold in pharmacists', and many people think of them as medicines. They are simply wines, of no special merit, to which have been added B vitamins or glycerophosphates or bitters. We have already seen that the B vitamins are of value to very, very few people, and the glycerophosphates to none; and the best that bitters will do is perhaps to help improve one's appetite. In other words, any benefit a tonic wine brings is due almost entirely to the wine it contains.

Of course, wine, when used in moderation, is one of the pleasantest items in life. Because of the alcohol in it, wine will help to improve appetite and digestion, will loosen one's inhibitions so that one talks more freely, and will help one to relax. All of this will be of value to someone who is *convalescing* from illness, or who is exhausted from temporary overwork, for instance; but it will be of no real value to a person suffering from an iron-deficiency anaemia, or a depression, or the earliest stages of a serious bodily illness – and who feels run down in consequence. Indeed, it may induce a feeling of false security, and delay that person visiting his doctor.

One should not, in other words, use a wine as a 'tonic' unless one is quite sure of the cause of the symptoms that have made one feel in need of a tonic. And if one is sure of it, and sure that wine would be appropriate, why take a *tonic* wine? Why not a straightforward table wine from France or Germany, or even England? (Yes, England, because some quite satisfactory, simple wines are made in this country from grapes imported from France; though the wine snobs wouldn't believe it.) For the same price as a tonic wine, one will get a table wine that is at least as good *qua* wine, and that is not cluttered up with B vitamins or glycerophosphates, which add nothing to its value. And one last point: wines are meant to be drunk before and with a meal, and in company. Don't start taking a wine – plain or tonic – or any other alcoholic drink, by yourself at eleven in the morning. If you feel like doing so, go and talk to your doctor instead. And tonic wines are alcoholic: never try and deceive yourself that they're not.

Before we end this chapter on tonics let us remember what was said at the beginning. Being run down can be due to any one of dozens of causes, some serious, some not serious at all. Each cause will need its own particular kind of treatment, so there cannot be just one 'cure-all' tonic that will benefit everyone who is feeling run down. And the vast majority of rundown patients should be seen by a doctor, who alone is able to decide what the cause of the condition is, and what its treatment should be. Often it is only a doctor who can provide the treatment.

If you are *positive* that the cause of your feeling run down is some simple personal factor in your life, then see that it is eliminated; and if you can't eliminate it altogether, try the effect of a holiday, or talking things over with a friend or a priest, of a glass of wine now and again, and of attention to the basic things of life, like sleep, food, and exercise. Don't expect a bottle of medicine to be any kind of substitute for these

commonsense steps. Remember that, even if a medicine is de
sirable, most patent medicine tonics, as we've seen, are of little
or no value, quite apart from the lay person's difficulty in
choosing the right one for his condition from among the few
different kinds there are. Let your doctor prescribe any 'tonic'
medicine that's needed.

Above all, if you are middle-aged, and perhaps the bread-
winner or the person in the family round whom the whole
household revolves (and that is usually the mother), don't say
to yourself that you can't spare the time to go and see your
doctor, or can't run the risk of him putting you to bed for a
week or so; and therefore you must take a bottle of tonic. It
may be that you are feeling run down or exhausted because
you are just starting with some serious illness, which your
doctor will probably be able to nip in the bud if you see him
straight away. Give him the chance to – and give yourself the
chance to be cured and made fit to go on being important to
your family for years and years ahead.

15

Travel Sickness, Sedatives, Anti-smoking Remedies, Aphrodisiacs

WE COME now to a mixed group of drugs for none of which could a place be found anywhere else in this book. The only other thing they really have in common is that they mostly act on the nervous system, or else on the mind. Certain drugs that are dealt with in other chapters also act on the nervous system (pain relievers, for instance, or 'pep' pills or certain cough medicines); but they were in groups of drugs that called for a section all to themselves. And of course, as for acting on the mind, most drugs owe some of their value to the effect they have on it – to suggestion, in other words. However, one section of the drugs dealt with in this chapter owe their effect almost entirely to suggestion. These are the aphrodisiacs. And the 'nervous system' drugs we'll deal with are travel sickness remedies, sedatives, and anti-smoking remedies.

Travel sickness remedies: they are certainly effective in a good proportion of people, and therefore useful; but they all have one snag in common – they can cause drowsiness. There's not much good in having a trouble-free plane journey back from the Continent if one steps out of the plane and drives one's car away – straight into the next world. Not everyone is made dangerously drowsy by these drugs; and even though one of them makes you drowsy, another of them may not. On the whole, however, unless you have had a few preliminary words with your doctor about it, or know from experience what effect it has on you, you're probably best advised not to take any one of the travel sickness remedies. If you do, be prepared for drowsiness and all its possible consequences.

Travel sickness remedies are of two kinds – those containing a hyoscine salt, and those containing an antihistaminic drug, usually either meclozine or cyclizine. No one knows exactly how these drugs work in preventing motion sickness. Although they are mild sedatives, this does not explain their effect, because more powerful sedatives, like the barbiturates, as well as most tranquillizers, have no effect on the condition. Probably they cut down the number of messages coming to the brain from the balancing organ in the ear. They are all much better at preventing motion sickness than at getting rid of it once it has started.

Hyoscine has a shorter action than the other two, but it also causes rather more drowsiness, and it is probably best kept for short journeys, lasting a matter of hours; meclozine and cyclizine being used when a journey is going to last for some days – a transatlantic crossing by ship, for instance. In the case of a short journey one can take these remedies half to one hour before the journey starts, but if the journey is to last some days, and meclozine, for example, is being used, one may prefer to start treatment with it up to a day in advance.

It should be realized that these remedies are not effective in *all* circumstances for everybody. If you cross the Great Australian Bight, for instance, in a gale, even your ship's captain may suffer from motion sickness, no matter what remedies he may have taken, and no matter how long he has been at sea And the use of a travel sickness remedy does not mean you can neglect other precautions. If you're travelling in a car, for ex ample, and are liable to travel sickness, ask the driver to go at a moderate speed, especially on twisting roads. When at sea, stay on deck in the open air during short journeys, if at all possible; and on any journey keep near the middle of the ship – half-way between bow and stern, in other words. And eat too little, rather than too much. (By the way, we now think meclozine and cyclizine are probably safe in pregnancy.)

Finally, no travel sickness remedy will affect the psychological element in the condition: if you start a long car journey by assuring little Jimmy (who's nearly always sick) that he isn't *going* to be sick this time, is he; and then let him see you putting a receptacle and a sponge beneath his seat; and then say he'd better not have that egg for breakfast, after all, as it might lie heavily on his stomach, mightn't it – well, don't expect, after such a brain-washing, that any travel sickness remedy at all will prevent little Jimmy being well and truly sick, and enjoying every minute of the commotion he'll cause. He'll probably start at the exact mid-point of your journey, the point of no return.

And now for sedatives – that is, drugs that will quieten your nerves, and, if taken in big doses, may help to get rid of an insomnia. Any drugs having this effect will, of course, be dangerous if taken in large amounts; and so practically all drugs of this type can be obtained only on a doctor's prescription. The best-known of them are the barbiturates. However, there are certain analgesics that have a mild relaxing effect, either alone or when taken in combination; and it is these that are contained in patent medicine sedatives.

The analgesics commonly found in such sedatives are phenacetin, salicylamide, and lactylphenetidin. The first two of these substances were discussed in Chapter 5. The third is simply a mild analgesic with no special virtues or vices. If one can't get to sleep because of some pain, then any one of these substances (or any other analgesic), whether taken in what the manufacturer calls a pain-relieving tablet or in what he calls a relaxing tablet, will be of value: it will help you to get to sleep. Of course, the cause of the pain should also receive some attention as soon as possible. In addition, even if no pain is present, the patent medicine sedatives may be of some value in helping you to sleep: phenacetin has a very mild relaxing effect, and the combination of phenacetin and salicylamide is said to have a rather stronger one. However, the action is still very mild, and if your insomnia is at all severe or if it persists more than a night or two, go and see your doctor.

Never be satisfied with taking these very mild sedatives night after night, perhaps in increasing doses: as we saw in Chapter 5, phenacetin can cause serious kidney damage if taken over a long period. And in any case, the sooner any but the mildest insomnia is tackled by an expert (that is, your doctor) the better: insomnia, like sleeping soundly every night for eight hours, is very often a matter of habit, and bad habits are very quickly established. Also, although a lack of sleep doesn't do any great harm, there may be some serious underlying cause for it – or less serious, like taking tea or coffee or a medicine containing a brain stimulant late at night. Let your doctor find out.

Are hot milky drinks any good for insomnia? – Some people are helped by them; others are particularly helped by a warm bed; others by five minutes' reading or by counting sheep. Whatever helps you to get a sound night's sleep is good, even though one needn't believe a tithe of what's said in the advertisements for milky drinks or electric blankets.

And now anti-smoking remedies. Those that contain drugs will usually be found to contain a substance called lobeline. This is a drug that has been known for a very long time, and in many ways its action in the body is similar to that of the nicotine that smokers certainly obtain from their cigarettes, pipes, and cigars. It has been argued that, because lobeline's action is similar to that of nicotine, one should be able to substitute it for nicotine, and so relieve oneself of addiction to smoking.

Alas! for this nice, tidy argument, things are not so simple. In fact, as we shall see in the next chapter, smoking is not simply a matter of nicotine addiction – which may, indeed, be relatively unimportant. And then, lobeline does not act in the body exactly like nicotine. And if smoking *did* simply consist of a powerful nicotine addiction, and lobeline *did* act like nicotine, all one would achieve by providing a lobeline pill would presumably be an addiction to lobeline pills instead of to cigarettes. Finally, and most important, tests of these lobeline anti-smoking remedies have produced no evidence that they are of any value.

And now aphrodisiacs. Apart from any intrinsic interest they may possess, one good reason for dealing with them in this book is that there are a few patent medicines that are sold as aphrodisiacs, however surreptitiously; and more important, that many very well-known patent medicines are believed by some people to be aphrodisiac, although their manufacturers certainly do not claim this property for them. Aphrodisiacs and patent medicines, in other words, are not poles apart.

The mere use of the word aphrodisiac is enough to make some people giggle and others hold up their hands in horror – the reaction depending on whether they are immature about sex (the giggles) or hypocritical about it (the horrors). The sexual appetite, however, is every bit as powerful and as normal as the appetite for food, and its satisfaction at least as pleasurable; so why should attempts to improve it when it is weak not sometimes be regarded as perfectly proper? If our appetite for food is weak, we soon do something about it. No reasonable person, speaking with a middle-aged man who has found his sexual appetite or powers on the wane, would want either to laugh at him or to censure him; and any person who would want to should conceal the fact – because he, or she, has something much more worthy of shame and of concealment.

It is not, of course, only middle-aged men (and women, if less commonly) who take aphrodisiacs, or consider taking them: old people do so; and young people as well, when their appetite for sex has become jaded, or when they imagine it should be keener. (Poor things, very often! Not realizing that too much sex is as sad as too little.) Also, let it be said that the fact of one sympathizing with many of these people does not mean that the use of aphrodisiacs has no moral implications, for it clearly has. What one can, however, ask for is a cool, rational consideration of the topic.

All right. Well, first a panoramic view of the aphrodisiac field. Beauty, of course, is an excellent aphrodisiac, though a vivid imagination is even better – perhaps fortunately, as there is never enough beauty to go round. Youth is the next best of aphrodisiacs, with variety close on its heels; and wine the next – though in moderation, for one must not fall asleep and merely dream. Dress (or its partial lack), gait, movement, and gesture, perfume, good food, pleasing surroundings, gentle lighting, and gentle music, the preliminaries in dalliance to love's final expression – all these too are powerful exciters of the sexual passion.

It is only when these 'natural', almost instinctively applied, garnishings fail that one turns elsewhere. One probably turns first, if one's own imagination has failed, to aphrodisiacal literature, or 'artistic' photographs; and both are, of course, available in profusion on most London bookstalls. And after the books there are certain films, and erotic paintings, and those sad decoys of a noble passion – what are called dirty pictures.

And what next? Well, apart from the tawdry and often sadistic salacities, whether performed privately or semi-publicly, to which one can buy admission in this and other countries, there are specific items of food, herbal remedies, and drugs. These are what most people mean by aphrodisiacs, and the number of them that has been recommended as aphrodisiacal is very large indeed. Among foods are almonds, curry, onions, oysters, anchovies, beef-steak, bananas, brains, caviar, celery, chocolate, bamboo shoots, spinach, radishes, eggs, mushrooms, tomatoes, turnips, crayfish, pheasant, quince, jelly, cockles, and figs. What risks we all do run!

Among herbal-type remedies alleged to be aphrodisiacal are wormwood, mandragora, basil, sage, paprika pepper, thyme, mint, fennel, marjoram, cinnamon, caraway, calamus, and juniper – a list that, if it has any validity, might make some of us gaze with a new interest at our herb gardens. And, lastly, among drugs that have been recommended are amphetamine, marihuana, Spanish Fly, cocaine, and yohimbine. Let us leave out of account the less commonly available items, like crocodile tails and lizard flesh; and the purely lunatic ones, like Queen

Bee jelly, which used to sell wonderfully in fashionable shops in London's West End.

What conclusion can one draw from this catalogue? If all these substances have genuinely been thought, sometimes over a period of centuries, to be aphrodisiacs, what is one forced to think? Surely that anything at all will very likely be aphrodisiacal if only you believe in it strongly enough; that most allegedly aphrodisiacal effects – like the impotence or boredom which they are desired to counter – probably arise from psychological influences. It is mostly in the mind, is sex; human sex at least. And thank goodness it is! – for otherwise Romeo and Juliet would be no more than a couple of copulating earthworms on legs.

The fact is that most of those who think of using aphrodisiacs need psychological help. Some gradual waning of the sexual powers comes with increasing age, as part of a general decay, mental and physical. In middle-age, however, it very often comes as a result of a depression (which may be difficult to detect) or some other mental disorder, such as an anxiety neurosis. And impotence or frigidity in youth, when not due to a neurosis, is nearly always accompanied by anxiety – an anxiety associated with rigid moral standards, or sexual ignorance, or excessive veneration of the loved one, or even plain doubts as to one's capacity to complete love's expression in a way satisfactory both to oneself and one's partner. And the right way, therefore, to deal with all these diminishments of sexual power must *au fond* be psychological. In some cases a little explanation and reassurance will be enough. In others treatment by a psychiatrist is necessary. But in practically no case is an allegedly aphrodisiac drug or food necessary, unless one would count as an aphrodisiac a mild sedative given to counter anxiety.

But might not an aphrodisiac be needed to enable psychologically normal people to indulge their sexual passions even more often than unaided nature will permit? No, for to wish for extremely frequent sexual intercourse is a sign of one of three things: serious mental illness, an intense but frustrated passion, and immaturity – most commonly the third. It is certainly not a sign of psychological normality, or of superhuman potency *pace* those immature American novelists who think it is. We are, all of us, much more of a muchness sexually than those ladies and gentlemen imagine.

The plain fact is that aphrodisiacs in the formal sense are practically never needed; which is as well, because hardly any drug or food is an aphrodisiac.

Let us consider the drugs that have been described as aphrodisiacal. The first of them is marihuana (Cannabis Indica, hashish, Indian Hemp, Mary-Jane, etc.). When smoked or swallowed, this drug produces a feeling of well-being, with hallucinations and some loss of self-control. It is a drug of addiction, though not strongly so; and has been used for centuries in the East, much as we in the West have used alcohol and tobacco. It is not aphrodisiac at all. Stories of teenagers or Hollywood stars going to reefer parties which end in wild sexual orgies may well be true; but any sexual actitivies will have occurred in spite of, not because of, the physical action of the marihuana. Of course, if people believe marihuana (or pickled cabbage or caraway seeds) are aphrodisiac, especially if they have to pay a lot for the marihuana, etc., and consume it in an atmosphere of secret conspiracy and anticipation, then, of course, sexual activity is liable to occur. But it should not be blamed on the marihuana, which, if anything, produces passivity in the people who take it. Marihuana is undesirable for various reasons, but not because it is aphrodisiac. It isn't in the least.

Yohimbine is another allegedly aphrodisiac drug, made from a West African tree. It almost certainly has no aphrodisiac action. Cantharides (Spanish Fly, Russian Flies) may have some aphrodisiac effect because the body gets rid of it through the kidneys and the bladder, which, like any other part of the body, are intensely irritated by contact with one substance it contains. As a result of irritation, sexual feelings may be stimulated, God having closely linked our sexual and urinary organs. However, it's all a little like sprinkling pepper on an inflamed area of skin so that one can get an increased satisfaction from scratching it.

More important – and quite apart from this kind of effect being likely to appeal only to ill or immature minds – Spanish Fly is an exceedingly dangerous substance, which has caused death more than once. That substance we just mentioned irritates much more than the urinary apparatus: it irritates the gullet and stomach when swallowed, producing difficulty in swallowing, and vomiting; later it irritates the bowel, producing colic and bloody diarrhoea; and it irritates the skin, if applied to it, producing huge blisters. It is, in fact, simply a very dangerous irritant to the body. Even a very small dose may have fatal results – quite apart from the fact that someone with vomiting and severe diarrhoea is not likely to harbour or to excite any sexual passion at all. Moral considerations aside, aphrodisiacs that may kill and that may, in the event, have an anti-aphrodisiac effect are hardly worth bothering about.

Other allegedly aphrodisiac drugs could be treated in this way, one by one. However, they all fall into one or two main categories. The great majority are in the marihuana category – that is, they are thought of as aphrodisiacs, but have no aphrodisiacal action at all. A small minority of them do have an aphrodisiacal action of sorts, but this is really a result of an irritation of the kidney and bladder – an irritation that may be dangerous or even fatal, either when affecting the urinary apparatus or when affecting some other part of the body. The names of this group will not be given here because some foolish people might be tempted to experiment with them. That of Spanish Fly has been given only because it is widely known and is much the most famous of them – undeservedly famous – and because, although not a strong aphrodisiac, it is a very powerful suicide or murder weapon: one way or another, anyone administering Spanish Fly to himself or someone else will very likely end up a corpse, not a Casanova.

And patent medicine aphrodisiacs? Well, a few of the allegedly aphrodisiacal herbal substances are present in various

16

The Commonest Drugs:
Alcohol, Tobacco, Tea
and Coffee

THERE ARE some people who will proclaim proudly that they
never take drugs – not even an aspirin for a headache. And a
few of them, when they come across a person who *is* taking a
drug, whether a patent medicine or a medicine prescribed by
a doctor, will tut-tut and talk about 'will-power', and about
how easily one can become dependent, and about what happened to an aunt of theirs in 1947.

The best way to deal with such people is to ask whether
they ever drink – beer or wine or whisky or anything else
alcoholic, including tonic wines. And if they reply indignantly,
'No, never', then one should enquire as to whether they smoke;
and if the answer is an even more indignant 'No', then one can
make practically certain of obtaining a 'Yes' by asking finally,
'But do you not drink tea or coffee?' Alcohol, nicotine, and
the caffeine in tea or coffee are, you see, all drugs, just as much
as aspirin or phenobarbitone or codeine are. And there is
practically no one who doesn't take one of them now and again.
A few words on these, the commonest drugs, may therefore not
come amiss.

The regular use of these drugs, at any rate in moderation, is
tolerated and indeed encouraged by our society. And of course,
in other societies there has been a similar tolerance to the use
of drugs like hashish, cocaine, and opium. 'The mass of men,'
said Thoreau, 'lead lives of quiet desperation.' And it is

because of such 'quiet desperation' that men have always sought
drugs that would provide solace or release, and have made
huge industries out of the production of such drugs, and important social and even religious occasions out of their consumption or particular phases of their production.

It may be said that, as just one example, the attraction of
wine to a connoisseur lies, not so much in the alcohol it contains as in the bouquet of the wine, in its flavour, in the aroma
it leaves behind on one's palate. Well, the attraction of a pretty
woman is greatly enhanced by any frills and furbelows she
may happen to wear; but it is her face and body that provide
the main attraction. Any man who doubts it should try admir-
ing the frills and furbelows in isolation – in a shop window,
say.

Let us look then at the actions of these three drugs, at least
one of which practically everybody takes. The caffeine of tea
or coffee is, of course, used as a drug in its own right. As we
saw in Chapter 5, it is very often combined with analgesics for
the relief of headaches (and it will relieve some headaches by
itself). In addition, it is used in one or two patent medicines for
the relief of asthma; and it is also available in patent medicine
form, as a tonic, simply for the slight 'kick' it will give one –
though most people prefer to get the kick from tea or coffee,
and don't call it a kick, especially not if they're maiden ladies
living in Bournemouth.

When used as a drug, the usual dose of caffeine is about 50
to 300 milligrams; and one cup of tea supplies between 50 and
100 milligrams, the same cup, if full of coffee, supplying rather
more. In addition to caffeine, tea supplies a very similar drug
called theophylline ('the divine leaf'), while coffee supplies one
called theobromine ('the food of the gods'). Caffeine's chief
action is, of course, that of stimulating the nervous system.
Because of this effect, caffeine will relieve fatigue, and act as a
stimulus to thought and conversation. People's performance
in various psychological tests has been shown to improve after
taking caffeine, although mankind's experience over the centuries had already supplied the best possible proof of the exis-

tence of this stimulating action. Taken to excess, of course, caffeine (or one of the drinks containing it) will, by the same token, produce restlessness, insomnia, anxiety, and trembling of the limbs. It is because of its stimulating action that caffeine is often combined with pain-relieving drugs, which themselves tend to depress the nervous system slightly.

What else does caffeine do? As we all know, it increases the amount of urine produced by the kidneys. So, of course, does a drink of water; and therefore a cup of tea has an effect on the bladder in two ways. Caffeine also increases the amount of digestive juice produced by the stomach; and this is why tea and coffee should be taken in moderation by people suffering from a peptic ulcer or from most other causes of indigestion. And lastly, caffeine improves the amount of energy that the muscles of the body can produce.

Caffeine is not a drug to which people become, in the strict sense of the word, addicted. It is not like cocaine or morphia: no one commits a crime in order to get hold of a cup of tea. However, we do become habituated to it, habituation to a drug meaning simply that, when one cannot get it, one does long for it. And it is as well for people of that superior kind with which we dealt with at the start of this chapter to remember the fact: they too, if they regularly drink tea or coffee, are to some extent dependent on the drug it contains. It is nothing to be ashamed of, but it may make them realize that we are all one flesh.

One final footnote on caffeine: William Cowper spoke of tea as cheering but not inebriating, what he had in mind obviously being the contrast between the effect of tea and of alcohol. The difference between them is, of course, a matter of common knowledge. It is curious, therefore, that the word 'caffeine' comes from the Arabic word for wine. Both wine and tea (or coffee) will, of course, stimulate conversation, but the ways in which they do so are quite different, as we shall see when we come to consider alcohol.

Let us first, however, consider that common accompaniment to tea or wine – tobacco, and more particularly the drug it contains, nicotine. Although the effect nicotine has on the body provides one of the reasons why people smoke, it is certainly not the only reason or the most important. In other words, cigarette smokers are not merely nicotine addicts. Nevertheless, nicotine is the only drug that tobacco contains, and to the expert eye there does seem to be at least an element of drug addiction in cigarette smoking. In addition, most of the bodily effects of smoking can also be produced by an injection of nicotine.

Let us look then at this substance which we use to kill insects and give pleasure to ourselves. A cigarette smoker who inhales will take into his body practically all the nicotine in a cigarette, which amounts to about three milligrams. A fatal dose of nicotine is upwards of forty milligrams; so that one packet of twenty cigarettes contains a good fatal dose. Of course, nobody smokes twenty cigarettes in two minutes, or even in two hours (not twenty whole cigarettes, anyway); and the cigarette smoker's body gets used to the effects of nicotine. He still, however, does take a lot of nicotine by medical standards.

And what exactly does nicotine do in his body, medically speaking? It stimulates and then depresses certain nerve ganglia. It also stimulates the nervous system in a particular way, which is not especially pleasant, and may indeed be highly unpleasant. What all this means to the person trying a first cigarette is nausea and perhaps vomiting, stomach griping, headache and giddiness and confusion, sweating and a feeling of faintness, and some disturbance of hearing and of vision. Of course, none of this happens to the practised smoker. His blood pressure goes up a little as he smokes and takes in nicotine, and his heart rate increases and the small blood vessels in his hands and feet close down or partially close down.

None of this is especially pleasurable. Nicotine does not stimulate the brain in the way that caffeine does. Nor does it quieten the brain, as alcohol or barbiturate drugs do. It does not make a person happy out of all proportion to the realities of his life, as cocaine and morphia do. Why then do cigarette smokers become so fond of tobacco? How exactly do they get the quietening, sedative effect that they say a cigarette gives them? The answer is that we do not know for certain.

Probably a part of the answer is that the smoker enjoys the stimulation to his mouth and throat produced by tobacco smoke: his pleasure is the same as the pleasure he gets from food, or that a baby gets from the breast. Indeed, some psychoanalysts think the cigarette smoker is perhaps seeking a mouth satisfaction that he did not enjoy as a baby, or did not enjoy for long enough.

Another factor is the whole 'ritual' of reaching for the packet of cigarettes, choosing and extracting one, tapping its end, reaching for a box of matches, removing one match from it, lighting it, putting one end of the cigarette in one's mouth, holding the match to the other – and inhaling. After all these preliminaries, often previously associated with pleasure, some pleasure is bound to be experienced – even though, for some reason, the cigarette has to be thrown away after the first puff.

And are smokers addicted to cigarettes or merely habituated to them? The answer depends on one's definition of these words. Certainly withdrawal of cigarettes from a confirmed and heavy smoker causes definite physical symptoms, and induces a craving for cigarettes in the person concerned, which may force him into wrong-doing in order to obtain some. What happened in cigarette-starved Europe in 1945 after the last world war showed how deep and powerful the desire for cigarettes can become; and, on the whole, it is difficult not to classify the heavy cigarette smoker as an addict.

However, those of us who do not smoke, and who perhaps become self-righteous towards our smoking friends and relations, should remember that the effects produced by any substance of addiction must be powerful, and must be of a kind that the addict finds to be in some way helpful in *his* life. If not, the addiction would not develop. Those of us who are not cigarette addicts may have, not so much wills that are stronger as personalities that are less sensitive or less perceptive than those of the smoker.

That plea for sympathy towards the smoker having been made, let it now be said that the case against cigarette smoking, irrespective of what benefits it may bring to any particular person, is overwhelmingly strong. Cigarette smoking is the main cause of lung cancer, and it is often a factor in causing or perpetuating such diseases as chronic bronchitis, peptic ulceration, and coronary heart disease. (Research has recently shown that smoking increases the stickiness of the platelets – or tiny particles – in the blood and makes the blood clot more quickly; and this may be the crucial factor in starting a blockage in the coronary arteries.)

The diseases mentioned can kill, and the fact of their association with cigarette smoking outweighs any benefit that cigarette smoking can bring. If you are in doubt, ask any one of the thousands of doctors in this country who have given up smoking in the past ten years. Why *have* so many doctors given it up? The answer is obvious; and lung cancer is now decreasing among doctors, whereas it is increasing among other people. Surely it is not only doctors who have a strong attachment to life.

And now for the third and most important of the drugs we take unashamedly in our living rooms – alcohol. Some people may think it strange to describe alcohol as a drug, but it certainly is one – an anaesthetic and analgesic drug. However, although it was used in the past as an anaesthetic (though not nearly as often as it should have been), and is still sometimes of value for the relief of pain, it is now used mainly for its psychological effects: as we all know, alcohol relieves people's shyness and social anxiety, makes them confident and talkative, and makes life seem brighter and its difficulties less dreadful. Taken socially in small-to-moderate amounts for these effects, alcohol is one of mankind's happiest discoveries. But taken uncontrollably in larger amounts, alcohol is certainly the curse that many teetotallers think it.

And which is it on the whole? A curse or a boon? Obviously the answer given will depend on one's personal experiences of the good and harm produced by alcohol, and on the particular scale of values one has. And the answer will differ in different places and at different times. Probably most people today would regard total prohibition as a preferable alternative to, say, the nineteenth-century gin palaces. Equally, faced with a community – and there have been and are some – where most of the drinking consisted of two or three glasses of beer or wine each day, most people would be opposed to prohibition. And in England today? Well, it is not the job of a doctor to moralize and legislate; but there does seem to be excessive drinking in this country today in two quarters – among some businessmen and among some young people. And the current advertising of alcoholic drinks appears to foster this excess in these groups. Some action to curb the excess probably should be taken.

And now let us consider alcohol, the drug. Alcohol is described by doctors as a depressant, even in small amounts, to the nervous system. Contrary to popular beliefs, it is not a stimulant at all. But then how is it that a glass or two of sherry makes so many people talk more freely and wittily? The answer is that they're usually not more witty, although those who listen to them, having had a drink themselves, often imagine that they are. The greater freedom in talking after alcohol – which is a real effect – is due to the action of the alcohol in depressing first the very highest parts of the nervous system, those involved in social inhibitions. The inhibitions are removed, and the person talks freely, smiles at people he hardly knows, says just what he'd do if he were Prime Minister, and so on. This is not stimulation, but destruction – a temporary destruction of part of the veneer of civilization, and one that may be very desirable after a long, tiring day, or after a meeting that has gone on for hours; but that is nevertheless a destruction.

Misconceptions about how alcohol acts in the human body are very widespread. There was recently a talk on the radio by a man who for years had had the job of going to the homes of people who had won large amounts on the football pools, and telling them of their good luck. Almost invariably, he said, they invited him to have a cup of tea, but never a glass of champagne: they wanted a sedative, he said, but not a stimulant. The fact is that tea is a stimulant, not a sedative, and alcohol (from champagne or any other source) is certainly a sedative.

Carefully conducted experiments reveal that even the smallest amount of alcohol makes people perform less well in various tests than when they are sober; tests of driving skill, for instance, or of typing, or of aiming at a target. Alcohol makes people less accurate or slower in such tests, and also slower in reacting to danger. The only exceptions are those few people whose performance when sober is affected by extreme tension and anxiety, and in them a *small* amount of alcohol may actually improve performance – and understandably so. The great majority of us, however, are made *less* efficient by alcohol, and this is the reason why, in the view of many doctors, including myself, one should drink little or nothing if one is going to drive shortly afterwards. Even a couple of drinks could, in a driving emergency, mean the difference between life and death for somebody. Unfortunately the same alcohol that impairs our skills also makes us unaware of what it has done, and even gives us a false confidence in our abilities.

What else does alcohol, the drug, do? It makes our vision and hearing less effective, and it makes us careless; in low concentration it stimulates the appetite and the secretion of stomach juices (but not in high concentrations, when it irritates the stomach); it makes us unsteady on our feet, and makes our speech slurring; it increases sexual desire but weakens its expression; it makes the kidneys produce more urine, and it helps us to go to sleep.

As we all know, an excessive intake of alcohol can make us vomit. This vomiting is probably not due to stomach irritation (though that is one extra causative factor), but to a high level of alcohol in the blood. Why? Because it can be produced simply by injecting alcohol into the blood stream from a syringe. It is fortunate that vomiting usually *is* produced by a certain high blood level of alcohol, because a level only a little higher puts a person into coma, and one that's a little higher again puts a person into the next world. People can, indeed, die from drinking too much on just a single occasion. Usually such people are drunk and take one further big drink without quite realizing what they are doing, and the extra drink is enough to raise their blood alcohol to a fatal level.

Alcohol is often taken to 'warm one up'. The 'warming up' feeling is due to two things: a burning sensation in the throat and gullet due to irritation by such spirits as whisky and brandy; and second, an opening up of the small blood vessels of the skin, which most alcoholic drinks, but particularly spirits, will produce after a few minutes. Once the blood vessels are opened up warm blood flows through them, and the chilled skin becomes warmer and feels warmer.

However, there isn't much point in feeling warmed up if, as a result, one dies a day or two later; and this is what has often happened. People who are going out into a very cold atmosphere take a drink first, their skin blood vessels are opened up, they feel warmer and go gaily out among the snow and ice, the blood vessels stay open, the blood in them is chilled, it circulates round their bodies, and so their bodies become chilled – and they die of pneumonia a few days later. The closing up of the blood vessels of the skin, with the consequent sensation of feeling cold, is a means of protecting the body from being chilled by a cold environment. Reverse the process with alcohol, and you're asking for trouble. It is, of course, quite permissible for someone who has been out in the cold, and is coming into a warm house for good – it is quite permissible for *him* to take a drink. It will make him feel warm more quickly than the warm house alone would; but he should avoid going out again – at least until the alcoholic glow has worn off.

And now for a few miscellaneous medicinal points about alcohol. A lot of people treat the early stages of a cold or 'flu by going to bed and taking a couple of aspirins and some hot toddy. There is no medical justification for the toddy, though there are other kinds. Second, never take barbiturate sleeping (or sedative) drugs after taking alcohol. Both barbiturates and alcohol depress the nervous system, and the two together seem to enhance one another's action. More than once a person has had three or four drinks late at night, has then gone to bed and, perhaps out of habit, has drowsily stretched out a hand for a box of sleeping tablets – and equally drowsily has taken half a dozen, instead of one or two. And that hand has never stretched out again. Never, never mix alcohol and sleeping tablets – or alcohol and travel sickness remedies.

Next, most people fail to realize that alcohol is a food, at least in the sense that it supplies energy calories. Indeed, it supplies more calories than the same weight of sugar or starch. This is why heavy drinkers are often heavy in other ways; and it is also the reason why they can sometimes get along while eating very little in the way of normal food. However, alcohol contains nothing but calories – no protein or vitamins or minerals or roughage. The cirrhosis of the liver that is common among alcoholics is probably due, not to an effect of alcohol in the liver, but to a lack of vitamins, resulting from the victim having lived for a long period on little but alcohol and slops.

As most people have appreciated, alcohol is quite rapidly absorbed into the body, except when it is taken very dilute or very strong. Most of the alcohol in the average drink is absorbed into the blood stream within half an hour. Absorption is, of course, slowed down by food; and is much quicker if alcohol is taken after a period of fasting. The body gets rid of a little alcohol in the breath and urine, but most of it is broken down in the liver (to provide calories); and we now know that the bodies of alcoholics *are* better able to deal with alcohol in this way than the bodies of teetotallers.

That is one reason why alcoholics need a much greater amount of alcohol than the average person to achieve the same degree of intoxication. Another reason may be that the alcoholic has simply learnt to take no notice of certain effects of alcohol that the normal person cannot but notice. By the way, I do not use the word 'intoxication' to mean being drunk:

intoxication, strictly speaking, begins with the very first sip of the very mildest sherry.

Disulfiram, the ethical drug that can be of value in stopping the alcoholic from drinking, interferes with the body's breakdown of alcohol, so that a substance called acetaldehyde (which normally the body can break down further) accumulates and causes flushing, palpitations, dizziness, vomiting, and collapse. If a person has taken some disulfiram, then the taking of an alcoholic drink at any time during the succeeding week may produce such symptoms; and of course, after a few experiences of them even the alcoholic will find that he has turned against his gin or whisky.

Although disulfiram is of some help in the treatment of alcoholics, there is no outstandingly effective way of dealing with them. Each victim has to be treated on his merits, with one or with a number of forms of treatment, which can range from disulfiram to help from that excellent organization, Alcoholics Anonymous. Notice the word 'victim' was used: the alcoholic is a sick man, and should be treated accordingly. People who treat him as though he were a moral outcast should be asked whether they treat people suffering from cancer in the same way – there is as much justification. And the fact that religious belief undoubtedly helps many alcoholics does not disprove the basic fact that they are sick people, who need treatment for sickness, not for sin. It is partly because of the moral slur attaching to their condition that many alcoholics will not come forward for treatment; and so there are many tens of thousands of unrecognized alcoholics in this country.

Alcohol has a few uses in medicine, apart from those that have already been mentioned *en passant*. In a seventy per cent solution, for instance, it is quite a good antiseptic for the skin and for instruments. It is used to harden the skin and to diminish sweating and itching in bed-ridden patients (and many years ago Scotch whisky, I have been told, was regularly used to harden the feet of hikers). In cases of severe pain, especially if long continued, alcohol is sometimes injected into whatever nerve is conveying the pain impulse to the brain – the nerve thus being destroyed. However, alcohol's main use, in medicine as in ordinary life, is to reconcile man to the world he finds himself in; and that is not such an inglorious use – it is, after all, one of the uses of those religions in whose names the alcoholic has sometimes been uncharitably condemned.

Of course, although the chief reason for taking alcoholic drinks is to experience the effect of the alcohol they contain, they do contain other things – pigments, whether natural or artificial, various essential oils and other aromatic substances. The importance of these is small in a drink like gin (consisting chiefly of alcohol and water plus some oil of juniper, an essential oil that increases the flow of urine and acts as a mild irritant to the urinary passages). It is of some importance in drinks like beer and whisky. And it is of considerable importance in the case of wines, and perhaps, to a lesser extent, of liqueurs.

The varying effects (especially the next morning) of different alcoholic drinks may be due to these extra ingredients. However, nobody is quite sure exactly what causes a hangover: an excess of alcohol is nearly always involved, but then people who drink too much have often eaten too much at the same time and smoked too much and gone to bed very late, so that other factors than drink may be important.

The best way to treat hangovers is a matter of dispute, even among doctors. Very few favour aspirin preparations (which are undesirable because they may further upset or damage a stomach that the alcohol has already inflamed); some favour vitamins, some a mixture of an analgesic with an antacid, some an amphetamine tablet, and some a good, hot, strong, sweet cup of tea. However, they all agree that much the best approach is preventative: don't drink too much. And if you find that you seem to be getting hangovers quite often, do go and consult your doctor, because you are not using alcohol, you are abusing it, and you are then sick and in need of expert treatment.

17

Patent Medicines in
the Dock

WE HAVE now looked in detail at the virtues and the vices of all the chief kinds of patent medicines, and at those of certain extra items like medicated shampoos and vitamin products (not to speak of tea, beer, and tobacco). And we have reached the final section of this book, perhaps the most important section, in which we shall take a much broader view of the patent medicine industry and its products.

We shall first – in this chapter – judge the patent medicines themselves, largely on the basis of all the medicinal information the reader has acquired so far. We shall then discuss the attitudes of doctors and pharmacists to patent medicines (attitudes that explain a great deal about their value or lack of value), and how those attitudes might change; and briefly consider the manufacture of patent medicines, and their labelling. Then we shall look at their advertising in some detail. And lastly we shall consider whether they should not be abolished, what forces gave rise to them, and what future there might be for them if they are not to be abolished.

In this chapter, then, we are going to weigh up the virtues and vices of the different groups of patent medicine, chiefly on the basis of their medicinal qualities. Of course, when deciding about whether to *buy* a particular product, one has to consider, not only the medicinal qualities of the drugs that the particular product contains, but also its price and perhaps the conditions for which it is recommended by the manufacturer. You may decide not to buy a product that is effective but very expensive; and if you are conscientious, you may make the same decision about a product that is advertised as benefiting some condition for which it is useless – no matter how good it may be for some other condition. So here, before we sit in judgement, is a little guidance on prices and manufacturers' claims.

Prices: the drugs in the vast majority of patent medicines are not patented at all, so that the maker of any one of them has no monopoly, and the price is therefore decided by what he can make the market stand. In fact, in the case of any particular broad group of preparations, some members are usually much better value than others. How can you discover whether a particular product provides the best value? Well, perhaps you already know which products are of much the same kind; and if not, your pharmacist will tell you (or you could work it out for yourself with the help of this book). Knowing the competitors and their ingredients – which are stated in the formulae – you can, by referring to one or other chapter of this book, compare the *medicinal* value of the various products; and you can find out at your pharmacist's or supermarket what all the products *cost*. Then, bearing in mind each product's medicinal qualities and its price, you choose the one that provides the best value for money.

And the conditions for which the manufacturer recommends his product? We have already spent some time here and there on this topic, and we shall spend a lot more when considering the advertising of patent medicines. We shall also mention it a few times in the present chapter, when deciding on the medicinal value of certain patent medicine groups, for to a considerable extent one can judge that only in the light of the claims being made for them.

However, we cannot hope to mention in a single book *all* the misleading patent medicine claims there are; and the reader can easily do some homework on this topic himself before making a purchase. If he is in any doubt about some claim being made by a manufacturer in an advertisement or elsewhere, all he has to do is to look at the names of the ingredients, discover in the appropriate chapter of this book what they do in the human body, and compare this with what the manufacturer is claiming. He will then be in a position, if he is so minded, to apply the small sanction of not buying any medicine for which dubious claims are being made.

And now let us make a start with our judgements of patent medicine groups by looking at external applications. The 'medicated' element in most medicated shampoos didn't do much good, we decided, though it didn't do much harm either. Deodorants and anti-perspirants, however, were an effective group of products with very few snags. Of the antiseptic soaps those containing hexachlorophene were the best of a not very impressive, though harmless, bunch. When used as they commonly are used in the average home, antiseptics and disinfectants probably are not particularly beneficial, except to the super-egos of house-proud ladies.

And then there are all the other items we apply diligently and hopefully to our exteriors: the rheumatic balms and liniments, which are reassuring and sometimes have an interesting smell, but don't really have much else to offer; the antiseptic ointments that aren't nearly as valuable for cuts and grazes as soap and water or the cuddle from Mother that usually accompanies their application; the ointments for skin rashes, which the manufacturer knows may be applied to any one of fifty different kinds of rash, so that they're not especially suited to any particular one; the acne preparations, which are quite useful but don't provide a sufficient treatment all by themselves; the eye lotions that may do a little good — and, like all these external preparations, don't do much harm. The exception to this catalogue of inoffensiveness was any preparation intended for the ear, because lay people should not put anything into their ears unless it's been ordered by their doctors.

Verdict on this group of 'external' remedies? 'Not Guilty', perhaps chiefly because many of them are at least innocuous. (In this chapter we are going to say 'Guilty' or 'Not Guilty' quite often, and by these terms we shall be meaning beneficial or not beneficial to the health of the people.)

Next, analgesics. Despite its effects on the stomach, there is no doubt that aspirin (the basis of most analgesics) is a highly useful drug. We could hardly get along without it. And yet (let those who believe in legislation and controls to make people virtuous ponder this), if aspirin had been discovered in the 1960s and a very wide-awake doctor had uncovered its defects straight away instead of – as did happen – fifty years after its discovery, there is little doubt that it would have been relegated by some committee or Government department to the limbo of drugs that were too dangerous to be released to the public. Indeed, it might have been banned even as a remedy to be obtained on prescription. It is only because we all know that for over half a century aspirin has proved valuable in almost every home that we can put its undoubted faults into proper perspective.

One cannot be so kind to most of the other drugs that figure in the various mixed analgesic preparations. Phenacetin, for instance, is quite a good pain reliever and a very mild sedative, but you will remember that it can harm the kidneys, affect the blood, and even cause headache itself. On the whole it is a drug we could do without. Codeine constipates people; but in the amounts found in analgesic mixtures (amounts that are controlled by law, not by the manufacturers), it probably doesn't relieve pain. Salicylamide has a very short action, and paracetamol not as valuable a one as aspirin, though both appear to be fairly safe. The caffeine in pain-relieving mixtures? It has a definite value and few drawbacks. And so what is the verdict on analgesics as a whole? Thanks largely to aspirin 'Not Guilty'.

What's next? The antacid indigestion remedies, which are almost all useful and harmless, though they should be taken for simple indigestion and not for a self-diagnosed peptic ulcer. And then we have that mixed bag of medicines for the stomach and intestines and the organs that go with them. The irrational combination of a bitter and an aperient, for instance: the bitter to improve one's appetite for food and the aperient presumably to jolly food along one's bowel before it can be absorbed into the body. The digestants, which practically nobody needs, and which, in any case, unless specially protected, are liable to be digested themselves by the stomach juices before they could possibly accomplish anything.

And then come the preparations in this group that are alleged to wake the liver up, when doctors know that the liver is very rarely asleep, and when their chief constituent is nearly always a strong purge which acts on the bowel, not on the liver at all. And lastly, we talked about the gripe waters, which may have a mild, useful effect on babies' colic; and about remedies for piles, which should be treated by a doctor and not with patent medicines. Verdict on this group? Again 'Not Guilty', chiefly because sales of the antacids are bigger than sales of all the other items put together, and practically all antacids are safe and effective.

However, the verdict on our next big group of products – the laxative group – is quite definitely 'Guilty'. And this is an occasion when one can reach a verdict only when one looks, not mainly at the products themselves, but at what the manufacturers say about them. A majority of laxatives, as we saw, are effective and fairly harmless if taken occasionally, when really needed. It is true that a few of them are quite unnecessarily violent in action; that liquid paraffin can leak from the anus; and that phenolphthalein can cause a skin rash. But these are the exceptions. What certainly can be criticized, however, is the fact that, encouraged by the manufacturers, people take laxatives when they don't need them, and will take them over and over again, thus causing a very great deal of harm. On the whole we'd be better off if most patent medicine laxatives were dumped in the Atlantic Ocean. 'Guilty' every time, the laxatives; though some of the guilt belongs to the Great British Public, as much as to the manufacturers.

Slimming preparations get the opposite verdict. This is because the most commonly used ingredient in them is methylcellulose, which is not particularly effective, but equally is not particularly harmful. They do, however, only just scrape through with the verdict of 'Not Guilty', for among the slimming preparations are some that are essentially nothing but laxatives. These are irrational, misleading in their claims, and wholly undesirable; and it is only because their sales are not big that they weren't allowed to swing the verdict to 'Guilty'.

And now remedies for the common cold. Ointments and aerosols don't do a lot of good, or a lot of harm. Inhalants are useful, thanks chiefly to the steam that goes with them. Nasal drops, sprays, and inhalers contain vasoconstrictor substances that close up the engorged blood vessels in the nose, but most of these substances carry certain risks that often outweigh their advantages. Simple analgesic and anti-fever remedies, mostly containing aspirin, are certainly useful for the common cold; but once they are mixed – as happens in the newest tablets and capsules for complete cold relief – with those vasoconstrictor substances, they become much less innocent, for they can then cause an undesirable rise in blood pressure. Another usual ingredient of these tablets and capsules is vitamin C. Probably neither vitamin C nor any other vitamin will help to cure or to prevent the common cold. Verdict on common cold remedies? It could, quite reasonably, go either way. Let the reader decide.

When we move on to cough preparations, there are so many defendants, and almost everyone of them contains so many ingredients, that a single comprehensive verdict is almost impossible. Cough preparations that are meant to be sucked do little harm, but probably most of any good produced by them results from the increased flow of saliva they cause. Among liquid cough medicines those containing cough suppressants or substances to open up the bronchial tubes do usually work fairly well, although most patients needing medicines of this kind should probably be in the care of a doctor. Cough remedies, in fact, range from those that are certainly effective but sometimes undesirable (as freely available patent medicines) to those that are not effective at all but are very pleasant to take. Verdict? Perhaps as this is a very complicated field, even for doctors, we should assume that, on the whole, the manufacturers have done their level best: give them the benefit of any doubt, in other words, and say 'Er – Not Guilty'.

There is, however, no doubt that vitamin preparations

should be pronounced 'Guilty', if not in a very loud voice. This is not so much because they do a great deal of harm: they don't – the cases of vitamin D poisoning that occurred among infants a few years ago were mainly the fault of the Government's expert advisers, not of the manufacturers of vitamin products. However, when one looks at the products in the light of what their manufacturers recommend them for, one is bound to say 'Guilty'. Broadly speaking, the manufacturers recommend them for all kinds of people and conditions, and yet the plain fact is that the majority of people in this country don't need extra vitamins at all, whether they're sick or well – they're getting plenty from their food. The fact that the recommendations of the manufacturers are often *sotto voce* or by implication does soften the indictment a little, but it doesn't alter it.

Another group that should be pronounced 'Guilty' – and this time in a fairly loud voice – is the group of so-called tonics. This again is not because of any great harm they do of themselves, but because, as they are put forward and taken as medicines that will help if one is feeling run down or fatigued or off-colour, they may result in certain people deferring a visit to a doctor when these vague symptoms are due to some serious disease needing early diagnosis and treatment. People with cancer or anaemia or early melancholia need a doctor's care, not a bottle of tonic.

A further criticism of patent medicine tonics is that, when the vague symptoms just mentioned are not due to anything serious, they can usually be made to go if the person affected can be led into a better understanding of other people or into working a little less hard or into having proper meals, but he may never consider such solutions if he is putting his faith in a tonic. Some of the tonics are nothing but foodstuffs in a highly expensive form, some contain 'nerve foods' that never yet made any nerve feel hungry, some contain yeast (which will *not* make you rise like a cottage loaf), and some contain iron – though usually not in really worth-while amounts, quite apart from the fact that lack of iron (that is, anaemia) should always be treated by a doctor. And tonic wines are really no different from any other wines: if you want alcohol, go to a pub and enjoy the company as well.

And finally, aphrodisiacs, which, in patent medicine form, are either useless little under-the-counter products or else are aphrodisiac only in the minds of certain of their customers; travel sickness remedies, which are a useful group of products but have the defect that they cause drowsiness; anti-smoking remedies, which don't work, any of them; and sedatives, which are very, very mild in their effects. Verdict on this mixed group? 'Guiltyish'.

But now what is the final overall verdict to be? There are two major points we should keep in mind before reaching it. One of them is the scale of usage of various patent medicines. There is no doubt at all that one's verdict would have to be 'Guilty' if one contrasted the *numbers* of separate patent medicines that are reasonably satisfactory with the *numbers* that are not – the dangerous, the harmful, the useless. But the percentage of items one could describe as satisfactory is much higher among the patent medicines that have a big sale than among those with a small sale; and one good analgesic, relieving tens of thousands of headaches every day, outweighs dozens of petty products that are useless but little used.

Second, a great many people, after reading the chapter in which laxatives were strongly criticized, will, without a thought, go and take – their usual laxative. And others, who are really needing beef steak more often, will swig some of their favourite tonic after reading in this book that tonics are without value. These people have a deep faith in their patent medicines, which isn't going to be shaken by what any crusading scientific doctor may say; and this is why the manufacturers of patent medicines can honestly swear, on the basis of the letters they receive, that their products do indeed have 'thousands of satisfied users'.

To be fair to the manufacturers, they are usually not aware that the benefits many such users get are purely psychological. One must, I think, be something of a sceptic, and have had some scientific training, and considerable experience to accept *readily* that a big proportion of people complaining of insomnia will go to sleep like a shot if you give them a 'sleeping' pill that consists entirely of sugar. This is what doctors call 'the placebo response', and it does take a lot of swallowing. The majority of doctors can swallow it, but not many other people.

Now, although I believe it to be mainly the result of much straightforward thought and hard work on the part of the manufacturers, and usually not of any sinister calculations on their part, it is certainly a fact that the advertising of many patent medicines, and the medicines themselves (their packing, their colour, smell, taste, and even consistency) are such as to induce the very psychological effects we've just been discussing. In other words, the medicines are what the pharmacist would call 'elegantly' presented – in every sense. And in my view, this is a real virtue, even though an insubstantial one.

The most sceptical of doctors, if he takes for his headache an aspirin tablet called, say, 'Miralgo' (and not just 'aspirin'), that comes from a tasteful, scientific-looking packet, that is beautifully finished and absolutely white, and that, for example, dissolves without bitterness in no time at all – the doctor will probably find his headache goes more quickly than if he had swallowed down the plainest of plain aspirin tablets from an ugly bottle. I have spent a lot of time on this topic because I think it very important to remember – and not only when *judging* patent medicines – that they often do good by psychological means, whether or not they also have a purely physical value as well.

And now what is our overall verdict to be? Most of you probably formed your own conclusions about patent medicines long ago, and this book won't have altered them at all; which shows how much we are governed by irrational factors. Though doubtless just as irrational *au fond*, I myself have *tried* to keep an open mind as we went along, and I have, in the course of writing this book, shifted my own provisional verdict now to 'Decidedly Guilty', now to 'Not Guilty by the skin of their teeth', and now to 'Somewhat Guilty'. However, my final verdict is going to be 'Not Guilty but very stupid. Put on probation'.

In what does the stupidity lie? Partly in the misguided 'information' the manufacturers often provide with their products or as an inducement to take them. And partly in the fact that patent medicines often contain very old-fashioned ingredients (sometimes in inadequate amounts), which, if they have any worth-while action, are usually less powerful, though correspondingly less dangerous, than the newer ingredients found in prescription-only drugs. Indeed, just about the most striking feature of patent medicines, when one looks at them *en masse*, is that in themselves they are neither very effective nor very harmful.

The prescription-only field is quite different: most ethical drugs today are powerful, and some of them can be dangerous for that very reason. Why this contrast with the patent medicines? One answer, of course, is that most of the conditions for which patent medicines are intended are minor conditions, which need mild remedies. In other cases there is a legal bar to the inclusion of a particular ingredient in a medicine that is to be freely purchasable. And in any case, no manufacturer is gladly going to risk his reputation by putting out, for general use, a medicine that is very powerful – and also, by the same token, dangerous.

However, even allowing for all these factors, it does often seem as though the many drug discoveries of the past thirty years – which have revolutionized the prescription field – have made much less impact on patent medicines than might reasonably have been expected. Cough medicines, antacids, aperients – the formulae of many of these, in the patent medicine field, any doctor would agree were old hat. And then there are certain kinds of patent medicine (reducing agents containing a laxative, ointments for the common cold, or six-ingredient skin ointments) that simply have no equivalents in the prescription field. If there were any, no doctor would prescribe them.

The biggest reason why there is this old-fashioned, stupid look to many patent medicines (and to much of the information that goes with them) we shall discover in the next chapter: it is crucial to any discussion of the industry's future.

18

Patent Medicines and
the Doctors

FOR A START, some facts. A survey conducted in a London County Council housing estate not many years ago showed that during a period of one month one person in every four took a prescribed medicine. But how many took a patent medicine during that same period? Two out of three. Indeed, a majority of people taking a medicine prescribed for them by a doctor also took a patent medicine. For every person who took a prescribed analgesic tablet thirteen took a patent medicine analgesic. For every one who took a prescribed laxative sixteen took a non-prescribed laxative. One in every four children was given a laxative during the month; and – most unpleasant feature of all – ninety per cent of these children were given the laxative, not because they *were* constipated, but to prevent them being constipated. And lastly, of all the medicines taken for haemorrhoids only fourteen per cent were prescribed, and of all the medicines taken for anaemia only a half were prescribed.

No matter how one looks at these facts, they call for study and for action; and a lot of the study and some of the action should surely come from doctors. So now what *is* the attitude of doctors to patent medicines? Well, a few doctors disapprove violently of patent medicine advertisements. Others, again probably in a minority, disapprove strongly of patent medicines being available at all, or of some kinds being available. But the mass of the profession merely disapprove of patent medicines, their antipathy being neither specific nor violent. It is none the less deep, and it is coloured with a very marked disdain. Why?

If pressed, most doctors will agree that it is reasonable for the average layman to keep a few simple medicines at home. And if a lay person should choose to have among those medicines some items of the patent medicine type (instead of the equivalent, when it exists, in standard form), the average doctor will merely shrug his shoulders at the thought of any extra cost involved. He approves of aspirin tablets, for example, under whatever name, being kept in the home, and of a simple cough medicine; of an antacid, and of a simple antiseptic cream; and perhaps of a trusted travel sickness remedy. Some doctors would go further and give their approval to an inhalant and perhaps an inhaler for the common cold, to an antiperspirant, and even to a mild laxative for occasional use.

Doctors give this limited approval, even though it is expressed half-heartedly, because they know the general public will continue to buy and use such remedies, no matter what doctors may say; because they know the average, sensible lay person can be trusted to treat those mild, short-lived symptoms of minor illness that afflict every family fairly often; and because they realize – at least some of them do – that, if there were no patent medicines, the increase in work for themselves would probably prove impossible to deal with.

At a deeper level, however, the medical profession does not really approve of patent medicines at all; and its disapproval and disdain take some curious forms. For instance, apart from an occasional glower, the profession's official bodies pretty well ignore patent medicines: one of the few occasions in recent years on which the British Medical Association even took cognizance of their existence was in 1949, when a special committee looked at their advertising. The Council of the B M A considered this committee's report, and in particular its suggestion that the following words should appear on every patent medicine wrapper, container, or label: 'If you do not obtain early and lasting relief of your symptoms, consult your doctor.' Now, of course, these words would normally be read only by someone who was going to take the medicine anyway, but the BMA Council rejected the apparently straightforward suggestion of its own committee (composed of doctors), and indeed described it as 'dangerous' – though in exactly what way it might be dangerous was not made clear.

A further suggestion, that the BMA should nominate a medical observer to attend meetings of the body concerned with the *British Code of Standards* relating to the advertising of medicines and treatments, was also rejected. And, finally, the committee had said in its report that 'Self-medication by the general public is a time-honoured habit'. The BMA Council changed 'time-honoured' to 'ineradicable'.

It is perhaps not the only habit that might be thought in-eradicable: all of this surely suggests that the attitude to patent medicines of the medical establishment, at any rate in 1949, was negative and unrealistic. One might have expected that the members of the Council – all of them doctors – would have shown a considerable positive interest in patent medicines, if only because, if they were not available, the doctors them-selves might well be overworked to the point of breakdown. Perhaps they felt that, if the habit really was ineradicable, no government would dare to abolish patent medicines, wholly or in large part; but in that case the doctors' duty to their patients should surely have dictated, not that they hold themselves aloof, but that they try to make this 'ineradicable habit' as safe and as conducive to health as might be.

Now why did those doctors in 1949 not argue in this way? And why do most doctors still not do so today? The profes-sion's attitude to patent medicines has, I suggest, a number of powerful causes.

First, doctors disapprove of people diagnosing their own ailments and then treating them accordingly. If the diagnosis is wrong, doctors say, the treatment will be wrong, and a minor disease may be turned into a major one. Or else, especially if a person has very great faith in a patent medicine, a dangerous disease may not be seen by a doctor until it is too late. This is a valid criticism. Patients who develop a cough, think it is just a 'touch of bronchitis' and treat it for some weeks or months with a well-loved cough medicine, may in the end turn out to have lung cancer. Other patients may treat a local skin rash with some unsuitable skin ointment, and before they know what has happened the rash has spread all over their bodies. Piles *may* be the first sign of serious internal disease.

However, one cannot always apply this argument because, if one did, lay people would have to be discouraged from *ever* treating themselves. Any treatment implies some kind of diagnosis. Thus the person who takes an aspirin tablet for a headache of a kind he perhaps gets every month or two is really saying something of this kind: 'I have a mild headache. I think that quarrel at the office has brought it on. Anyway, I am pretty sure it is not due to meningitis or a brain tumour or high blood pressure. And I think it is a suitable kind of headache to be treated with aspirin.' And when one takes an antacid tablet or powder, one is really saying something like this: 'I have some heartburn and nausea and stomach fullness, probably because I had too much to eat and drink at that party. My symptoms, I believe, are not due to a peptic ulcer or to cancer, and it is quite all right for me to treat myself with some of this antacid.'

Now, as we have already indicated, most doctors would approve of home treatment in these two instances. In other words, the medical maxim that lay people should not treat themselves with home remedies on the basis of having diagnosed their own complaint is not invariably applicable, even in the eyes of doctors. When it would appear highly probable to any reasonable person that a complaint is a minor, short-lived one, most doctors would agree that home treatment is permissible. In the case of obviously serious or chronic complaints, or when there is any reasonable possibility that symptoms have a serious or chronic cause, then naturally such treatment is quite out of place.

It should be added that, to some extent, the objection doctors have to lay people making any kind of diagnosis of their own complaints arises from the old-fashioned wish that a minority of doctors still have to keep all things medical a closely guarded secret; and the extent to which this attitude can be carried was well illustrated by one of the fellow doctors with whom I discussed patent medicines while writing this book. He said he had no objection to lay people using patent medicines, but he would object strongly to any layman being given enough knowledge about drugs to be able to decide that, of all the headache relievers, *Bloggo* would suit him best, and of all the indigestion remedies *Peppo* was the right one for him. What this doctor was saying was that he would object to people being helped to make a *rational* choice of a patent medicine; though apparently he would not object to their making an irrational one. I found his attitude incredible.

Anyway, a second reason why doctors are ag'in' patent medicines is that, until about forty years ago, doctors themselves had no effective treatments for the majority of illnesses, apart from that minority of ailments that could be put right by means of an operation. The doctor was no better at curing than the patent medicine vendor. All the doctor could do for most seriously ill patients, by and large, was to diagnose exactly what was the matter – and he usually did that with considerable skill – and then to provide sympathy and coloured water until the patient died or recovered or became reconciled to the fact that he had a chronic disease for which nothing could be done.

A doctor, of course, had other and important functions: he would advise on health, he would bring babies into the world, he would splint fractures, and always he would give kindness and understanding to his patients. And quite apart from all these benefits he brought to the patient, he had a skill in diagnosis and in other ways that had cost him years of expensive training, and he had a social position to keep up; and therefore, for his own sake (not to speak of that of his patient), he had to defend himself on his one really weak front – that of treatment. If the majority of people knew what he acknowledged in his heart – that he could really do very little for them when they were seriously ill – would they continue to go to him as often as before, even when he could be of help? What would be the good of paying for a very clever diagnosis, if the disease was going to kill one anyway in six months? And why not take some patent medicine or some herbal remedy, if the doctor's medicine was really no better, and indeed was quite often identical with such nostrums? The patent medicine manufacturer (particularly as he could beat the big drum whereas the doctor's only corresponding weapon was his bed-side manner) was the doctor's serious rival when it came to treatment. And so the doctor of fifty years ago – whose bottles of medicine, to do him credit, were usually harmless, and in which he did have *some* faith – would bitterly attack the vendor of nostrums, whose remedies were often not harmless at all.

This attitude, which was once appropriate and understandable, is now quite out of date. Today's patent medicine manufacturer is in no genuine sense a rival to the doctor. Quite apart from the fact that there is a great shortage of doctors, which will persist for many years, the doctor today has a range of powerful drugs with which he can hopefully attack most serious diseases. He hardly needs his bedside manner (and so many younger doctors aren't bothering to cultivate one – to the distress of their patients). Everyone knows about antibiotics and cortisone and insulin, and how effective they are. And most of the new and powerful drugs can be obtained only on prescription: the patent medicine manufacturer is not free to put them into his products.

The basis for the old antagonism, in other words, is gone; and yet it persists anachronistically among the doctors. Perhaps the fact that, broadly speaking, the new drugs have been discovered, not by doctors, but by the same drug industry that provides patent medicines – perhaps this riles the doctors. But in fact their rivals today are not the patent medicine manufacturers, but the chiropractors and the naturopaths and so on, whose systems of treatment are quite different from that of orthodox medicine (not just pale reflections of it), and might therefore be looked upon as valid alternatives to it.

There is some simplification in all this. What has just been said applies as far as any thinking, informed person is concerned – the typical reader of this book, for instance. Such a person does know that today's patent medicine manufacturer is tagging along in the wake of medicine proper – that any drug *he* can provide the doctors can provide better. However, many patent medicine manufacturers keep the formulae and the exact mode of action of their products as quiet as possible, often because there's nothing very exciting to say about either. And alas! the cloak of strange scientific potency their products wear is thought by some simple people to be, not a mere disguise, but the genuine article. They believe, these people, that for almost any prescribed medicine there is a real alternative in patent medicine form. To what extent awareness that this attitude is present among many simple people is a factor influencing doctors in their continued enmity towards patent medicines is not easy to say.

The third reason why doctors dislike patent medicines is that they are closely associated with one of the most terrible words in the medical vocabulary – advertising. As everyone knows, doctors are liable to be struck off the *Medical Register* if, in the hope of attracting patients, they in any way advertise their knowledge or skill, or, on occasion, even their mere availability. This is a right state of affairs for any profession, and particularly for one concerned with illness and death. However, because doctors must not advertise for patients, and because the vast majority of doctors go to great pains never to appear to be indulging in any kind of 'puff' at all, many of them think that almost *any* kind of advertising is bad. And of course, patent medicines *are* very widely and forcefully advertised. However, the crew of an oil tanker cannot expect pipe smokers on land to share their attitude towards matches.

Another, lesser element in this aspect of medical antipathy towards patent medicines is the fact that doctors, perhaps more than any other group of men, are both concerned to discover truth and confronted with the many varieties of deceit in which men indulge and with the consequences of deceit. Advertising men, to put it at its kindest, are concerned to present a product in the best possible light, and the truth, or bits of it, often tend

THE DRUGS YOU TAKE

to disappear along the way. The exaggeration, the artistic
licence, the gloss, the desire to jostle people into spending
money – all the common and understandable characteristics
of advertising men and their advertisements are foreign to the
doctor. However, not all its faults can alter the fact that advertising is as integral a part of the selling of any article in our
economy as a stethoscope is of a doctor's equipment.

The fourth reason for the doctors' antipathy is that they
rightly believe the main, and usually the only, motive of the
patent medicine manufacturer is the profit motive. Doctors do
not like to think of people making money out of ill-health.
There is some lack of logic in this: doctors themselves, of
course, make a living out of ill-health, and there are some men
in the medical profession, often most able men, for whom the
money motive is a very powerful one indeed. Also, some patent
medicine manufacturers do, in fact, temper their commercial-
ism with something that approximates to the doctor's conscience.

And then, if money could not be made out of patent medicines, who on earth *would* provide them in our free, money-
orientated society? The state might conceivably do so; but if
there was only one kind of pain-relieving tablet, and two kinds
of cough medicine, and all patent medicines had the same
'National Drug Service' labels, and there was no advertising –
it is conceivable that then the doctors would have even more
work to do than they have now. They are nevertheless repelled
by the idea of businessmen trafficking in health for money.
The word 'trafficking' is one some doctors would use, and it is,
of course, calculated to rouse one emotionally.

One last reason for the antipathy is this. Doctors know that
seventy or eighty years ago the majority of patent medicine
firms were 'rackets'. Grossly extravagant claims were made for
products that were useless or harmful. And the same is still
true of a few firms – mostly the small, hole-in-the-corner ones.
However, doctors tend to shut their eyes to the improvements
that have certainly appeared in this century, particularly in the
last two or three decades. What helps perhaps to blind the

doctors to the new respectability of many patent medicine firms is the recollection that in the eighteenth century doctors used themselves to put out patent medicines of the worst type. The great John Hunter, for instance, one of the founding fathers of British medicine, did so. It takes a long, long time to live down that kind of activity, especially in one's own eyes; and of course, one tends to be allergic to any suggestion of it in others.

Lest it be thought that all or most of the reasons doctors have for disliking patent medicines are spurious, let it be said here that there are various other important reasons for their attitude, all of them valid: patent medicines, doctors say, are often taken quite unnecessarily, or over a very long period, and people are induced by their advertising to think of them as harmless and as essential to good health. However, these various important and real defects in connection with patent medicines will fall to be considered in some detail a little later, in the context of patent medicine advertising; and they are not, in my view, the most important factors determining the doctors' attitude.

The element that, in fact, chiefly underlies the doctors' attitude to patent medicines is the distaste they feel for commerce – the antipathy the professional man feels for the businessman. The doctor is afraid of being 'contaminated'. There was never much justification for this kind of antipathy, apart from snobbishness; and to foster it now is to carry into the twentieth century an attitude that was almost jejune in the nineteenth. Scorn for business is a middle-class foible this country can no longer afford. In any case, many doctors will admit in private that, in this computer age, some of the purely technical expertise and the drive of the modern businessman would do the profession a world of good.

Ought the doctors to change their attitude? Well, first, however big the artificial gulf – and indeed the real one – between them and businessmen may be, can the doctors afford *not* to try and bridge it today? This is an age of enlightenment: people will not tolerate what they conceive to be sectional, obscurantist attitudes, opposed to the general good. They want patent medicines to contain the best possible drugs, and they want to know the truth about drugs in general. Where should they turn, if not to the doctors?

Secondly, as we shall see later on, there is a very serious shortage of doctors today: the profession simply cannot afford to reject any kind of ancillary help, however difficult the initial liaison with the helpers might prove to be.

Thirdly, have doctors not some *moral* duty to stretch out a hand to the businessmen in the drug industry? Think of some of those figures with which this chapter started: most people taking a doctor's medicine also taking a patent medicine, thirteen times as many people taking a patent medicine pain reliever as were taking a doctor's pain reliever, nearly a quarter of all children being dosed with laxatives *just in case* they got constipated. If we assume patent medicines are here to stay, for the doctors not to start doing a great deal more than they are at present to put matters to rights would seem to be making professional dignity and outmoded attitudes a substitute for the study and action that is called for in the interests of their own patients. The fact that some of the reasons for the doctors' antipathy and disdain are valid – this is one of the strongest reasons for intervention.

It is, indeed, concern for their dignity, for the often effete forms of medicine, rather than for the vigour of its substance, that has been responsible for many of the troubles that have afflicted doctors in this country in the last twenty years: the field of patent medicines is one in which the profession could take an enormous step forward.

But what am I suggesting doctors should do? Two things. First, they should try, both in an organized endeavour and as individuals in the course of their daily work, to increase the amount of relevant health education they are giving to their patients. For instance, they should try to get it generally accepted, in the context of home medication, that most people don't need laxatives at all, and that suspected anaemia should always be treated by a doctor. There are a hundred similar lessons to be taught.

And then, as it seems quite reasonable for people to treat most of their headaches and other small aches and pains with a patent medicine analgesic, doctors should be prepared to tell their patients which patent medicine analgesics are desirable and which are not – those, for instance, containing phenacetin. And the same for cough medicines and antacids and so on.

Doctors recommend publicly advertised medicines? Yes, why not? Which is the more important, people's health or un-real ideas about professional dignity? People are taking patent medicine analgesics, and will continue to do so (with the ap-proval of doctors), and can do harm to themselves if they take the wrong one. A patient with a peptic ulcer, for instance, is probably best advised not to take those patent medicines that contain ordinary aspirin. Why should a doctor not say so, face to face with his patients, naming the suitable and unsuitable brands if necessary? The pharmacists can do that, someone will say. But the doctor cannot opt out of such an important sphere. And it is no disparagement of pharmacists to suggest that a doctor's word usually carries more weight. In addition, patent medicines, rightly or wrongly, are often bought else-where than in a pharmacist's, but each one of us has a family doctor.

It may be asked how, if there is a shortage of doctors and the profession is overworked, they are to find the time for all this education of patients. The answer is that it would not take such a lot of time, and it would soon, in fact, begin to reduce the doctor's work load. It would save time, not consume it, in the long run.

Of course, many doctors are doing just what has been sug-gested – recommending to their patients certain safe and valu-able patent medicines, either openly or tacitly, warning them against the dangers of inappropriate or excessive self-medica-tion, and so on. I am suggesting that this should become recognized as a proper course for *all* doctors, and should be recommended by their various professional bodies. But then wouldn't the doctors be bombarded with literature on patent medicines? Perhaps they would, as we still live in a free and

capitalist society. But they've been bombarded with literature
on prescription-only drugs for years: they have survived it,
and they are as free to throw any literature in the waste-paper
basket as the manufacturers are to send it.

The second, and perhaps the most important, way in which
doctors could help to ensure that the patent medicine colossus
operates fully in the interest of the people's health would be
for them to see that all drug firms had access to expert advice,
and for those doctors who *are* concerned with drug firms to
provide detailed and considered advice on patent medicines,
and to do so wholeheartedly, in the knowledge that they were
providing a valuable service that had the approval of all their
professional colleagues.

In my view, many of the defects of patent medicines and
the faults in their advertising spring from the almost complete
divorce there is between doctors, who know about drugs and
illness, and the businessmen, who know about manufacturing
and selling. Some of the smaller firms are not only without any
source of medical advice, but would be alarmed by any suggestion that they should seek help from a doctor. (And yet from
whom else should they seek it?) Others get advice now and
again from the local G.P. – who is usually, no doubt, a well-
meaning man, but who cannot hope to give the same quality of
advice in the field of drugs as could Professors of Medicine or
of Therapeutics. It is medical men of that calibre who should
be retained as consultants by the patent medicine firms.

Now, of course, such men do act as consultants to some of
the bigger drug firms. (Indeed, some of the most distinguished
medical men in the country are retained by them.) And nearly
always these firms also have a full-time doctor, or even half a
dozen full-time doctors, working on their products. However,
it is not usually the patent medicine products they or the consultants work on: it is the ethical products, those your doctor
will prescribe, the 'respectable' products. It is a statement based
upon experience that the consultants and the 'resident' doctors
will fight shy of a firm's patent medicine products; that because
of this the salesmen concerned with the patent medicines are,

in turn, reluctant to approach them; and that on occasion there is not merely a failure of communication between the two groups, there is coolness or even antagonism.

Apart from those firms, mostly large, that make both patent medicines and ethical medicines, there are some firms that make only one and some that make only the other kind of product. And it is of interest that the bigger of those making only ethicals do nearly always have full-time medical advisers, whereas the bigger of those making only patent medicines practically never do.

In some of the big, dual-purpose firms the situation often becomes absurd. A doctor in such a firm will spend weeks arranging for tests of, or writing literature on, a new prescription-only drug that, when it is available, may be used in no more than a few thousands of patients, perhaps with some not very serious complaint. But ask such a doctor to help in improving the formula of a patent medicine, or even to 'vet' an advertisement for it, and he will begrudge five minutes spent on such a job. And yet that patent medicine may sell to millions of people, and its total potential for good and ill be enormously greater than that of the prescription-only drug.

The present medical consultants and advisers in the drug industry, plus any extra doctors that might become involved if my suggestion were accepted, would not total more than two or three hundred altogether, but they would make a contribution to health out of all proportion to their numbers. However, there will be no extra doctors, and the present ones will probably not alter their attitude, unless the rest of the profession gives them some encouragement. Will it? I think it well might, for the medical profession is in a time of crisis, and could therefore be willing at last to accord some kind of recognition to an industry that is probably supplying people with more tablets and bottles of medicine than are prescribed by all the doctors in the country.

It is in part because so few doctors have been prepared in the past to help patent medicine manufacturers that, as we noted towards the end of our last chapter, any advice the manufacturers provide in connection with patent medicines is often hopelessly out of date, while the formulae of many patent medicines corresponds with medical thinking of forty, fifty, or sixty years ago – or even earlier. The drug revolution of the last forty years has hardly affected some manufacturers at all, particularly the smaller ones; and yet it should have made *some* impression, even though many of its products are not suitable for inclusion in patent medicines. Indeed, although the manufacturers have their share of cupidity and other unpleasant qualities, their chief fault is probably ignorance; and they certainly do not deserve all the blame for it. That verdict of 'Not Guilty but stupid' reflected on doctors to some extent, as well as on manufacturers.

Of course, not all of the responsibility for the present state of affairs rests with the doctors. Many manufacturers would be uneasy at the prospect of letting a doctor have anything whatsoever to do with their products, and others would be horrified (justifiably because of the nature of their products). In the event, however, once co-operation was established, the manufacturers might be pleasantly surprised by the doctors, most of whom, once their interest is truly engaged, are realists, aware that the world does not live on bread and honey. One might even see an extension here of the process, unexceptionable in some countries, but a novelty in this one, that in recent years has given the highest executive positions in one or two drug companies to men who are medically qualified. What more natural? And yet how rare it is!

What other difficulties in the way of liaison might there be on the manufacturers' side? Well, it should go without saying that, for all their ignorance of the workings of the human body and of drugs, the manufacturers are a very astute group of men. Astute enough, for instance, to know that, although a doctor may regard the ingredients of a particular patent medicine as old-fashioned or useless or even dangerous, the general public may have a different view. Indeed, a manufacturer will often leave the formula of a patent medicine unchanged even when he must know it could, by any reasonable standard, be improved. *Must* know? Yes, sometimes, because on occasion the very manufacturer who puts out a patent medicine that has an out-of-date formula (which makes it popular, even though it isn't understood) is sometimes also putting out a prescription-only product for the same condition that has a completely different and much more up-to-date formula.

Occasionally the manufacturer could plead that two quite different factories and groups of personnel were involved; but there is little doubt that in some of these cases the manufacturer simply has a double standard. One should not condemn him out of hand when the sales of his old-fashioned, over-the-counter remedy may be very high, and when he strongly suspects that the sales of an up-to-the-minute replacement would be very low, at least at first. (His shareholders are always ready with an up-to-the-minute replacement for him.) He has to live. The important point to note is that he is certainly astute enough to start making changes just as soon as the general public has been educated into wanting them, and the doctors are sitting at his boardroom table.

We come back, in other words, to our original conclusion: that the medical profession has a double responsibility – first, to educate and guide the general public, and second, to advise and prompt and push the manufacturers. This chapter has been written because I believe that the medical profession probably has more power (and a greater duty) than the manufacturers or the general public or even than Parliament to shape the patent medicine colossus into a modern, fully responsible, and fully effective guardian of the public health. And a colossus it is, however many doctors may wring their hands at the thought. Let it at least be a beneficial colossus with a medical brain to it.

19

Pharmacists, New Legislation, Labelling

ANY COMING together of the medical profession and the patent medicine industry, such as we discussed in the last chapter, will take some little time; and its fruits will take longer again to appear. However, we already have in existence a body, most of whose members are doctors, that is acting as a filter to the introduction of new patent medicines that have no proven value or that are dangerous. This is the Dunlop Committee on the Safety of Drugs, a body that was set up after the thalidomide disaster. Submission to it of details of proposed *new* patent medicines (it is not primarily concerned with old ones) is a voluntary matter although all members of the Proprietary Association of Great Britain – the patent medicine business association, to which most manufacturers belong – have said that they will submit such details.

However, highly important though it is, the Dunlop Committee is essentially concerned with something negative – that useless or dangerous remedies never get on the market. The kind of liaison I have suggested as desirable between doctors and manufacturers would add a positive aspect to this: it would ensure that those remedies that *did* get on to the market were the most valuable and the safest that could be devised.

The Dunlop Committee and its permanent staff have been very busy indeed since they started work on New Year's Day, 1964, and they have not yet been able to take a retrospective look at the vast majority of patent medicines which were already on the market at that time. However, such a retrospective survey, though it would involve a great deal of work, would very quickly effect a big improvement in patent medicines. I have little doubt that the Committee would order laxative reducing agents, for instance, off the market; and direct that, as just one example, the advertising of those products that are alleged to wake up one's liver should not mention the liver at all. A similar improvement could, of course, be achieved more painlessly if the doctor-industry liaison I have suggested were to become established; but failing that, the Dunlop Committee will doubtless in time take a long, hard backward look.

Another desirable function the Committee (or some other body) could carry out if the requisite machinery were available would be to 'vet' patent medicine advertisements to ensure that, for those products to which it had given its approval, advertising claims were, in fact, the same as had been mentioned in the original submission to the Committee. As we shall see in Chapter 21, a completely new body may be needed to deal with patent medicine advertising, and it could usefully carry out this policing function on behalf of the Dunlop Committee.

One final point about the Dunlop Committee: it seems likely that, in the comprehensive drug legislation that it is known the Ministry of Health intends to introduce before long, submission of proposed new products to the Committee will be made compulsory, as it should be. Indeed the Dunlop Committee as such will quite probably vanish, only to be reborn a moment later with its powers a good deal wider than at present.

This new drug legislation will probably contain two or three other important elements that will have an effect on patent medicines. The first concerns the conditions under which patent medicines are manufactured, and the standards to which they are made. Those readers who remember the brief descriptions given at the start of this book of pharmaceutical manufacturers and their premises will not be surprised to hear that, in the author's own experience, factory conditions do, in fact, vary from those that would not disgrace a hospital operating theatre to those that would not be tolerated in the average kitchen. It is likely that, under the new legislation, some system of inspection and control of manufacturing premises will be introduced: at present there is no control at all. However, whether the ultimate control, in this and other ways, should be exercised by the Minister of Health is very much in dispute: he is, after all, the chief purchaser, through the National Health Service, of the pharmaceutical industry's products.

As a corollary to control of premises, the standards to which drugs are to be manufactured will probably be laid down in the new drug legislation. From time to time one reads of a public analyst who has examined tablets of a particular drug obtained from half a dozen separate manufacturing sources, and has found perhaps three of them to contain less of the drug than they should. This defect in quality is usually due, not to any wickedness on the part of the manufacturers, but to a poor system of laboratory control in the factories concerned; and this slackness should certainly be remedied.

The ultimate effect of this legislation will probably be to eliminate the careless and the unhygienic firms and to leave only those firms that, in every sense, have a genuine stake in the patent medicine field. (Alas! small firms will probably go under too, and the difficulties in the way of starting a new drug firm will be greatly increased.) Most of the firms remaining will have laboratories, not only to control the manufacturing processes, but to carry out research for new drugs, and to develop from such new drugs products suitable to go out to the general public on free sale. It is only if it possesses laboratories of this kind that the firm will be able to make the advances that the public has a right to expect.

Usually, of course, research on new drugs for patent medicines goes hand in hand with – or, more often, is a by-product of – research on new prescription-only drugs; but this is as it should be. Nowadays a drug is usually, if at all, introduced in patent medicine form only after it has been employed for some time as an ethical drug; so that most of its faults have become known long before it is freely available. Such restriction should be compulsory.

One very important figure in all this – in the research laboratories, in the control laboratories, in manufacture – will be the industrial pharmacist. Why hasn't the pharmacist been mentioned before in this chapter? Why wasn't he mentioned with the doctors? Because there is no uniform attitude to patent medicines among pharmacists, as there is among doctors. Many of the sales managers, and production directors, and managing directors of pharmaceutical firms are pharmacists – as well as many of the laboratory personnel. But equally some of the sternest critics of patent medicines are to be found among pharmacists, some of the critics even being employed in the industry. This range of opinion is what one might expect in a body of men, most of whom are half business-men, half professional men. Although it should not need to be mentioned after what has already been said in this book, no criticism of pharmacists is implied when they are described as half businessmen. Their difficulty arises from their being part business, part professional men: both roles are perfectly respectable, but their combination creates difficulties. For instance, in a retail pharmacist's, his professional half may disapprove of a particular patent medicine, but his business half knows that, if he does not offer it for sale, his income will suffer. However, pharmacists are currently engaged in coming to major decisions on this topic, so no more will be said about it here.

But wasn't it being suggested in the last chapter that doctors should throw themselves into the affairs of patent medicine firms, and that more of them should become directors of such firms? Might they not become similarly schizophrenic? Well, the professional medical adviser to such a firm need not be, and usually is not, in any sense a businessman, whereas a pharmacist sales manager certainly is. And the percentage of doctors who might become 'business' directors of drug firms is extremely small – say, at best, no more than fifty or a hundred doctors out of the tens of thousands of doctors there are in this country. There would be no danger of the profession of medicine becoming half commercialized.

One matter affecting pharmacists that will probably receive a mention in the new drug legislation is the type of shop in which patent medicines may be sold. At present about half of the total volume of sales takes place in pharmacies, and half in other types of shop; and the new legislation will probably not alter this radically, although a system of inspection of all shops may be introduced.

Many pharmacists would like to see all or most patent medicines sold only in a pharmacist's; and they would justify this restriction on the ground that only a pharmacist (apart from doctors) knows of the danger of drugs, and is therefore able to give sound advice to would-be purchasers, and to control the sale of medicines properly. This is true, but, as regards the great majority of purchases of patent medicines in a pharmacist's today, advice is neither offered nor asked for nor desired. (In some other countries the pharmacist plays a very big part in health education, but pharmacists in this country are in two minds as to what extra commitments they should assume in this field.) There is something to be said for the sale of a few drugs – quite apart from drugs that are obviously dangerous or liable to misuse – being restricted to pharmacies, but in this imperfect world many patent medicines, perhaps most, can quite safely be sold elsewhere. And apart from anything else, as they *are* now being sold elsewhere, the British public might not take kindly to any marked restriction unless there was some very good and obvious reason for it.

There is one other matter needing attention on which pharmacists certainly have something to say, and that will figure in the new drug legislation. It is the matter of the formulae that patent medicine manufacturers put on labels. There is a legal obligation to provide the formula of such a medicine; and the Pharmacy and Medicines Act of 1941 lays it down that, when an ingredient is in either of the two official drug publications – the *British Pharmacopoeia* and the *British Pharmaceutical Codex* – the name used in the formula shall be the official name. (And then the ingredient must come up to the official standard in quality.)

The names used for other ingredients are usually the accepted scientific or trade names. However, what all this means in practice is that many names are in Latin, and in abbreviated form at that; and in fact, the formulae are almost meaningless to the man in the street. In any case, the official or accepted names of drugs are not always used when it appears that they should be.

There are two reasons why there is much to be said for using the ordinary English names for drugs (when they have such a name), as well perhaps as the Latin names. First, we are living in an age of enlightenment: ordinary people expect, in all sorts of spheres, to be told facts in plain English, and rightly so. And in practice, more and more doctors are telling their patients what drugs they are receiving and why. A great many pharmacists, however, appear to want to keep the general public in ignorance of almost everything concerning drugs. This is a rather old-fashioned attitude, perhaps justified when practically no drugs were of any value to a sick person, but quite out of place when there are dozens of useful drugs available to humanity. Perhaps the pharmacists are wanting to preserve the *mystique* of pharmacy, but they are running the risk of being ignored or of being regarded as old fuddy-duddies.

My own view is that it is not only sensible but right that on most occasions most people should know the truth and the whole truth about the drugs they are receiving. And incidentally that truth, as provided on the patent medicine label, should include information on any untoward effects of the drug, and on any special precautions to be observed when taking it.

A second reason for using plain English names for patent medicine labels (and one that everybody would support) is that a person who is allergic to a drug may know it only under its English name. For instance, a person who knows he is sensitive to aspirin may not recognize this substance under its alternative official name of 'acid. acetylsalicyl.'; and so may, in all innocence, take a tablet containing aspirin, and suffer a severe reaction. And, allergy aside, who wouldn't prefer 'peppermint oil' to 'ol. menth. pip.', 'dried yeast' to 'cerevis.

ferment, sicc.', or 'liquorice extract' to 'Ext. Glycyrrh.'?

Indeed, whether it is by design or accident, so very special-
ized are some of the names at present appearing in patent
medicine formulae that not even a doctor or pharmacist could
claim to recognize them at once. Confusion can also result
from the amounts of ingredients being stated as percentages
and not as the actual amounts by weight per dose. Percentages
may sometimes be used for convenience, as in the case of ointments, but it is surely desirable to keep such usage to a minimum. On occasion, for instance, when one works out what a
certain percentage of an ingredient really means, one discovers
it means a dose suitable for a mouse, not a man. A small mouse
at that, very often.

And lastly, when a manufacturer is listing in his formula
both the truly active ingredients (those that matter) and those
that are simply meant to hold the tablet together or make the
powder run smoothly or make the medicine smell nice, he
should indicate which is which – by listing them under the two
separate heads of 'Active Ingredients' and 'Inactive Ingredients'. What often happens at present, whether or not this is the
manufacturer's intent, is that six or eight substances are listed
in a formula (though perhaps only a couple of them are active),
and the simpler purchasers of the medicine think it must be
very powerful indeed if it has so many ingredients in it.

An ingredient of a patent medicine that is inactive or present
in an absurdly small amount is sometimes included, not because the manufacturer wishes to deceive or is trying to econ-
omize, but because it was first suggested seventy years ago by
the manufacturer's grandfather (or, as often as not, by his
grandmother). Nobody has given it a moment's thought ever
since – apart from the man who's been putting a pinch of
whatever-it-is into the tablet-mixing machine every week for
the past fifty years. And anyone who doubts that, in this computer age of ours, such a thing could happen, had perhaps
better turn back to the descriptions of individual firms in
Chapter 1, and start reading all over again.

*   *   *   *   *

Since the above was written the Government has published a White Paper outlining proposed new drug legislation; and all the necessary legislation is being debated in Parliament in 1968. Most of the proposals are not politically controversial, and it therefore seems likely that the legislation Parliament passes will correspond very closely with the suggestions in the White Paper. Its full effect on the British patent medicine scene will not, however, become apparent until the 1970s.

Here, in so far as it affects patent medicines, is what the White Paper has to say. There are to be statutory safeguards in relation to toxicity testing and to the assessment of drug safety – in other words, the present voluntary Dunlop Committee procedures *will* become compulsory. There is also to be control of the quality of drugs, of their distribution and sale, and of their labelling and advertising.

A lot of new work will be involved for the Minister of Health, and so a new body, the Medicines Commission, is to be set up to advise him on matters of policy and principle, and on the various expert committees that will be needed. It will also take over responsibility from the General Medical Council for publishing the *British Pharmacopoeia* (a volume laying down standards for many drugs).

Licences, to be issued by the Minister, will be necessary for the manufacture, importation, or marketing of drugs, and for drug wholesaling; and certificates will be needed before clinical trials of new drugs can be carried out. Licences may be refused or suspended, one of the expert committees being first consulted by the Minister if a technical point is raised. Appeal in the High Court on point of law will be possible.

Although this all sounds formidable, the aim, says the White Paper, is to achieve the same flexibility and even informality that has existed up to now in the work of the Dunlop Committee on drug safety.

The sale of drugs is not to be confined to pharmacies, though the drugs that may be sold elsewhere will be prepacked items to be listed by the Minister. It seems likely that most of today's patent medicines will figure in the list. There is to be control of hygiene and cleanliness in relation to the keeping, transport, and use of drugs.

As regards the labelling of drugs the inclusion of certain items of information will be compulsory. In particular, any needed warnings or precautions will have to be included; and misleading labels or leaflets will be prohibited.

There are also proposals in the White Paper affecting the advertising of drugs, and these will be discussed in Chapter 21.

Finally, the White Paper envisages sampling of drugs at all stages of manufacture and distribution, the right of entry and inspection, the right to have books and documents produced – and indeed all the powers needed to ensure that the purposes of the legislation are met.

The provisions of this proposed, wide-ranging legislation are certainly the most radical in the field of drugs for some decades. Some of them were anticipated earlier in this chapter, and their likely effects considered; but it is difficult to forecast what the other effects will eventually be without knowing just how the new legislation is to be administered.

The exact role of the Medicines Commission, for instance, is uncertain. The White Paper envisaged the Commission as being an advisory body, appointed by the Minister and in the last analysis not really independent of him. The Sainsbury Committee, whose report on the prescription-only side of the drug industry appeared shortly after the White Paper, also recommended the setting up of a Medicines Commission, but the Sainsbury version of this body, though financed by the Minister, would be independent of him except in licensing matters, and would have power to enforce its regulations. It would also have wider powers than the White Paper's Commission.

However, this and other uncertainties will soon be resolved by debate or experience. And they do not affect the main import of the new legislation, which is that the world of patent medicines should be very greatly improved during the next few years.

20

Controls on Advertising
of Patent Medicines

IN THIS and the next chapter we shall consider what is probably the most important single aspect of patent medicines – the one that comes first to most people's minds, the one that critics of the industry get hottest under the collar about, the one that makes use of some of the best brains in the drug industry. I mean, of course, the advertising of patent medicines. And if you're in any doubt as to its importance, here are just a few figures about such advertising for one recent year.

How much do you think different manufacturers spent on advertising their analgesic products – those containing aspirin, phenacetin, and so on? More than £500,000 was spent on each of two such products, and not much less on each of three others. In a single year.

A good deal less was spent on laxative advertising, although on three well-known brands of simple 'dose-of-salts' aperient a total of well over £600,000 was spent. Three leading antacids had nearly £100,000 more spent on them, while the three leading medicated shampoos also accounted together for more than £600,000 of advertising money.

In case these figures are so big that they mean very little to you, let us compare them with what some other quite different advertisers spent in the same year. A top brand of petrol and oil accounted for something over £1,000,000, a little more than that was spent on the advertising of a single detergent. However, the cost of all the advertising of the British Motor Corporation was only about £400,000, and of British Railways only about £700,000. There were, in fact, at least three patent medicine manufacturers who spent substantially more on advertising than did British Railways. Or, to provide another comparison, very much more was spent on advertising analgesic products alone than on advertising milk.

On the advertising of one vitamin product more than £200,000 was spent; and about £150,000 on that of each of another two. On the advertising of a single balm more than £100,000 was spent. On each of two tonics over £250,000 was spent. To spend £50,000 on the advertising of a product was small stuff, and £20,000 a year was chicken feed.

These, remember, are the figures for a single year's expenditure in the United Kingdom. We are certainly, in other words, in the realms of very big business. And we must beware of two kinds of prejudice. The first springs from the belief that the advertising of medicines, even the simplest, should be treated completely differently from the advertising of other products; the second from a belief that all advertising is bad.

Well, first let us agree that the advertising of medicines is *something* of a special case. Special because, when they are sick, people are usually more gullible than when they're well; and because most people know very little about the workings of the human body or of drugs, whereas we all know, for instance, whether or not we like the taste of an advertised food, or the cut of an advertised item of clothing, or whether that advertised holiday in Spain turned out to be worth the money. The advertising of medicines is special also because medicines can be dangerous, because matters of life and death and pain *may* be involved, because in actual practice there have probably been more abuses in such advertising than in any other kind of advertising.

However, we must not therefore imagine that patent medicine advertising is unique in all respects. After all, women can be very gullible about clothes or beauty products as well as about patent medicines. People know very little more about petrol or detergents, and the way *they* work, than they do about drugs. And motor cars cause more deaths than drugs do.

So, while the advertising of patent medicines *is* special, it is not all that special. It is, however, because many people do regard it as unique that a minor transgression in advertising, which would excite little comment if Scotch whisky or paint were involved, is quoted *ad nauseam* when it's a question of a patent medicine.

The second source of prejudice is an anti-advertising bias, which seems to be present in most people today, even including many of those who work in advertising. I am certainly not competent to defend the role of advertising in a free economy, and this is not the place for such a defence. In any case, most readers are probably tired of hearing of the importance of competition between products, the importance of the customer knowing that they are available, and all the other pro-advertising arguments that some Sunday newspaper economists spend much of their time playing tiddly-winks with.

I would, however, make one point: what people seem most to resent about advertising is the gap between the promise and the reality – between, in other words, what the product does and what the advertisement says or implies it does. Now it does seem to me that, gross deceits aside, resentment of this kind is quite out of place, because everyone knows that 'promise, large promise, is the soul of an advertisement' – of every advertisement. If it is reasonable to blame an advertiser for having made a product seem bigger, more colourful, more effective than it really is, then it is reasonable to criticize politicians for most of the promises they make, poets for nearly all their figures of speech, and young ladies for wearing make-up.

Exaggeration of virtues, playing down of faults – these are common human characteristics, and, so long as no big, misleading lies are told and everybody knows the rules of the game, their appearance in advertising shouldn't shock anyone, least of all politicians (who regularly profess to be shocked). Some of the puffs are in contravention of the various advertising codes, but many offend only the tender susceptibilities of some critics of advertising who think it should tell the truth, the whole truth, and nothing but the truth. The real difficulty arises, not in making all advertisements read like instructions on how to make a model aeroplane (any move to secure that would mean an end to all advertising), but in deciding when the forgivable puff ends and the really dangerous or undesirable deceit begins.

Well now, having looked briefly at the scale of patent medicine advertising, and reminded ourselves of two kinds of prejudice, let us look, as dispassionately as may be, at what means have been devised to ensure that patent medicine advertisements *are* reasonably truthful, not liable to arouse fear, and so on. The answer is a very complex *voluntary* network of codes and committees. At the centre is a document called *The British Code of Advertising Practice*. This lays down a series of 'do's' and 'don't's' in connection with advertising, and in particular has a whole section (more than half the code) dealing with the advertising of medicines and treatments. This forbids, among much else, any claim to 'cure' an ailment, any mention of diseases that call for medical attention, any misleading or exaggerated claim, any appeal to fear, any offer to diagnose ailments by post, and the offer of any slimming treatment that might do harm. In addition, it specifies by name dozens of conditions for which products must not be advertised. (This is in addition to diseases such as cancer, public advertisements for the treatment of which are already forbidden by law.) And finally, the preamble to the *British Code* states that it is 'intended to be applied in the spirit as well as in the letter'.

The British Code of Advertising Practice (which, incidentally, occupies six quarto pages) first appeared in 1962, but the section dealing with medicines and treatments first appeared in 1948 when, it may be remembered, the late Mr Aneurin Bevan was Minister of Health. That section grew from an even earlier code drawn up by what is probably the most important single body subscribing to the medicines section of the present *British Code* – the Proprietary Association of Great Britain, or the P A G B, as it is commonly known. This is essentially a business organization, which has as its prime object the protection of the interests of its member firms – that is, the patent medicine manufacturers. Not all such manufacturers belong to it, but most of the big ones do; and the P A G B's own *Code of Standards of Advertising Practice* first appeared in 1936 – and is still published today in a revised form. Curiously enough, the current edition of the P A G B Code forbids its members to advertise products for the treatment of cancer, epilepsy, tuberculosis, diabetes, and Bright's disease – although any public advertisement for such a product has, in fact, been illegal for the past quarter of a century.

Another very important body that subscribes to the current *British Code of Advertising Practice* is the Advertising Association, which represents the interests of all those people who are connected with advertising – newspaper and periodical owners, manufacturers, advertising agents, independent television companies, and so on. This association publishes a series of leaflets, supplementary to the *British Code*, on the advertising of particular groups of products – laxatives, vitamins, etc. Its leaflet on 'Advertising for slimming' (its own title), for example, states that the *British Code* forbids advertisements for laxative reducing pills. This leaflet appeared, however, only in 1963, whereas the dangers of such products were known to doctors long before that. (And at least one such product was still being made available to pharmacists recently; though needless to say, responsibility for this cannot be laid at the door of the Advertising Association.)

The Association has a number of offshoots. One is the British Code of Advertising Practice Committee (commonly known as the C A P Committee, for short), which is concerned with keeping the *British Code* up to date, and is the final court of appeal for interpretations of the code. Then there is the Advertisement Investigation Department Committee (the A I D Committee) with two sub-committees. This is the body concerned with investigating what are alleged to be fraudulent or undesirable advertisements, with advising members of the Advertising Association on the desirability of particular advertisements, and with helping both the C A P Committee and the third of the Advertising Association's offshoots – the Advertising Standards Authority Ltd.

The Association appoints the chairman of the Authority, and he in turn appoints its members. Individuals or organizations can complain to the Authority about particular advertisements, and it will have the matter investigated, and, if necessary, issue a public statement. (Its address, for anyone who is interested, is: 1 Bell Yard, London, W C2. This is also the address of the Advertising Association.) The Advertising Standards Authority was intended to be a kind of advertising equivalent of the Press Council, but it certainly does not seem to have achieved that stature yet; and indeed, there have been signs that the Authority and the Advertising Association – which originated it but from which it is supposed to be independent – do not see eye to eye over what constitutes independence.

As well as the P A G B and the Advertising Association, *The British Code of Advertising Practice* is accepted by a variety of bodies – the Independent Television Companies Association, the newspaper proprietors' business associations, and the bodies concerned with the interests of advertisers and of advertising agents, and of firms dealing with posters, screen advertising, and direct mail advertising. And various of these bodies, like some individual newspapers, have expert consultants, usually medical men, to whom they can refer proposed advertisements for an opinion.

Because television advertising can be so influential and because there is such a lot of it, the Independent Television Authority was instructed in the 1964 Television Act to draw up its own code governing advertising and to see that it was complied with. And so in July of that year, after consulting the Postmaster General, and its own Advertising Advisory Committee and Medical Advisory Panel, the Independent Television Authority published its own Code. In fact, as regards the advertising of medicines and treatments, it accepted that part of the *British Code* that dealt with them, but added to it a few extra rules of its own.

A patent medicine manufacturer who has a new product must, of course, submit its formula, etc., to the Committee on Safety of Drugs; but he will also take the formula, the proposed claims and advertisements, the product pack, and any leaflets that he wants to use with it along to the P A G B secretariat, who will advise him as to whether or not he is proposing to contravene any rule in the *British Code*, any relevant legislation, etc. And he will take the same step in connection with a new advertisement for an established product.

If his advertisement is for newspapers or periodicals, it will next be scrutinized by the appropriate copy committee – that is, the committee set up by the newspaper owners or the periodical owners, acting jointly, to look at the wording and illustrations of new advertisements ('copy' simply means the words in an advertisement.) It will again be scrutinized by any individual newspaper in which he wants his advertisement to appear; and, of course, at any stage the manufacturer may find himself involved with the C A P Committee or one of the many other bodies we have been discussing.

If a television advertisement is contemplated, then both the secretariat of the Independent Television Authority and the Copy Committee of the Independent Television Companies Association (the Programme Companies Association) will scrutinize the script of the proposed commercial, and later will scrutinize the filmed commercial itself.

All this may sound wonderful; and indeed, when one reads what some of the people who operate this system have written about it, one would suppose it impossible for any advertisement that was not completely truthful to get through the net. It is not possible to be sure to what extent advertisements are, in fact, modified or turned down by the scrutinizing bodies, for they do not make their findings public (and they are fully entitled not to). However, my own experience and investigations lead me to think that a considerable proportion of advertisements are, in fact, modified as a result of the application of this control system. More important perhaps is the question of whether all those that should be modified are modified; and to that my own answer is 'No'.

Two major and two minor comments on the system itself would seem to be justified – for those readers who are still awake. The first major comment is that, although committee-making and committee-sitting are popular British ways of whiling away the time, the number of committees involved in the control of advertising, especially patent medicine advertising, is extremely large, and their functions seem very often to overlap. This cannot make for efficiency, to put it at its mildest. Various relevant committees and associations have not been mentioned at all, and yet the majority of readers must have been completely flummoxed by those that have been listed on the last few pages – as the writer himself almost was. (Indeed, in one leaflet on advertising the Advertising Association itself got so confused that, when listing the complete range of interested committees, it mentioned the same committee twice over under slightly different names.)

Second major comment: there is one characteristic common to practically all of the committees – they are set up or controlled by organizations whose members have a financial interest of some kind in advertising. They may be manufacturers who hope the advertisements will sell their products, or newspaper owners who get paid for the space taken in their papers, or television people whose income in the end comes from the advertisers who buy time on the little screen: the end result is the same – they have a financial interest in seeing that advertisements appear. It may be said that, at the moment, there are, for instance, far more advertisers wanting to buy television time than there is time to sell, or that there are also newspapers that can afford to pick and choose among their would-be advertisers. It none the less remains true that a man should not be asked to be judge in a cause to which he is a party.

It is not being claimed that the individuals involved are not doing their job quite conscientiously – for most of them probably are. (And indeed, a few of them have no direct contact with advertising.) Or that no improvement in patent medicine advertising has been secured in the last twenty years, for that is clearly not true. What is being claimed, however, is that men who are dependent on advertising for their livelihoods or their profits should not be the main judges of the acceptability of advertisements; and that further improvements could probably have been secured by a single scrutinizing body, composed of men who had no financial interest in advertising at all.

And now for the two minor comments. First, some of these committees, etc. have no power to apply sanctions against transgressors, others have. However, one very rarely hears of them being applied; and it may be suspected that, as in the average club, a member of some particular organization has probably to commit some most heinous advertising offence before he is expelled.

Second, there is something of an inbred air about most of the various bodies discussed: the same old names crop up time and again. Here is just one example of the thinking behind this state of affairs. When preparing this book, I asked the chairman of one of these many committees whether he would regard it as proper that a doctor who was acting as a medical consultant to his committee (that is, providing a neutral expert opinion on advertisements) should also be acting as medical consultant to a firm whose advertisements the committee might scrutinize. Answer? The chairman said he could not see that there was necessarily any objection at all to this. And he seemed to mean it. Many readers may take a different view, as I certainly did. Perhaps there are not a lot of committees really. Perhaps there are only one or two. And perhaps that is the trouble.

21

Advertisements – their Defects and their Better Control

ACCORDING TO some patent medicine advertisements, Gilbert and Sullivan's gondoliers must have been hard put to it to *find* a young lady with a pair of sparkling eyes, let alone take them. Why? Because the young ladies they met did not have the benefit of the vitamins, laxatives, and tonics we enjoy today; and only those products – or so it seems from their advertisements – can make one's eyes sparkle, give one abundant good health, etc., etc., and then only if taken regularly.

How much in claims of that kind is mere verbiage and puffery, not to be taken seriously, and how much is untruth or exaggeration that misleads and that calls for an antidote? How widespread *are* claims of this kind? And how are they to be recognized? Well, in a sense practically all of this book has been answering these questions, especially the last one. Each time you have read a statement that substance A has a particular action in the body you have really been invited to compare that statement, which is the truth, with statements made about substance A (under whatever proprietary name) in an advertisement or leaflet. Still more, when you read in this book that substance B certainly does *not* have a particular effect, you can be pretty sure that the effect has been claimed, or is being claimed, for substance B in some advertisement somewhere.

Nobody can really say how widespread are untruths, exaggerations, etc. in patent medicine advertisements, for no organization has the specific duty to find out. Indeed, probably no organization is fully equipped to find out: they all lack money or personnel or motivation. This is quite understandable when one thinks of how each day dozens and dozens of newspapers and magazines are published, most of them containing patent medicine advertisements. And yet it is most desirable that we know how widespread are transgressions of the *British Code* (and indeed of other standards that may be thought appropriate), for without such knowledge one can only guess at the effectiveness of the present methods of control, and suggested improvements to them can be only rough and ready.

Having made that proviso about our relative ignorance of the size of the problem, let us look at some patent medicine advertising that exemplifies it. For obvious reasons the names of individual products cannot be mentioned; but what will be written is based on a study of some hundreds of advertisements for all kinds of product, and only such camouflage has been used as was thought necessary to protect a product or a manufacturer from recognition.

Well now, first, there are some provincial newspapers and smaller periodicals that regularly contain patent medicine advertisements clearly contravening the *British Code*. Indeed, many of these advertisements – for anything from aperients to 'aphrodisiacs' – would make some readers' hair stand on end, and would reduce the average doctor either to white-hot rage or to uncontrollable laughter. They are usually small advertisements, any illustrations in them are crude, and they contain a mass of words providing untruths, half-truths, incitements to fear, and so on – plus what advertising men would call a good hard sell of the product. Such advertisements are certainly not confined to the less respectable publications: one periodical that is otherwise the soul of respectability regularly contains a number of advertisements of this type.

What is the explanation? In the case of some very small publications and minor products it may be that there is ignorance of the *British Code* or of its provisions. More commonly, the publication concerned and the manufacturer simply do not belong to those organizations whose members have agreed to abide by the code – the P A G B in the case of the manufacturer, and the Periodical Proprietors' Association in the case of the periodical. In these latter circumstances no organization, not even the Advertising Standards Authority, has any power to apply any kind of sanction in order to stop the advertisement(s) continuing.

These, however, are the small fry: the big manufacturer advertising in the national daily newspaper or on television is probably capable of much more harm. Yet judgement in his case is often difficult. This is recognized in *The British Code of Advertising Practice*, which says in its preamble that 'The Code is intended to be applied in the spirit as well as in the letter'; and in its television equivalent, the *Independent Television Code of Advertising Standards and Practice*, which says, 'The detailed rules set out below are intended to be applied in the spirit as well as the letter'.

Now, although it is sometimes difficult to establish beyond all cavil that in a particular advertisement an advertising code is not being observed in the letter, it is unfortunately ten times more difficult ever to *prove* it is not being observed in the spirit. Any judgement in this field must often be a judgement of intent more than of words and phrases. It is often the implications of an advertisement, the undertones, the general drift that are found to be objectionable: every word of it, every phrase may be acceptable, but somehow the totality is not.

All right. Roughly how common then are contraventions of the advertising code? My own judgement is that there are some contraventions of the letter and a good number of contraventions of the spirit of the advertising codes by the big advertisers; though fewer on television than in newspapers, and far fewer in the latter than there were fifteen or twenty years ago. In addition, not all of these contraventions are mere harmless puffs, such as we mentioned in the last chapter. Some of them are capable of doing harm and should be stopped. And often the advertiser is aware, fully or partially, of what he is doing.

However, even though practically all breaches of the codes should certainly, in my view, be rectified, I believe that we should not be particularly *offended* by many breaches of their spirit, or by certain breaches of their letter, for that matter. We should not, in other words, adopt an attitude of moral censure towards the advertisers concerned. It is, after all, hard enough for most men, when their livelihood is involved, to abide by the letter of any restrictive rules governing their activities: it is next to impossible for them to abide by their spirit – that is, to support the rules in their hearts, particularly when the rules sometimes seem to them to be a shade removed from reality. How many motorists truly respect parking regulations, as distinct from abiding by them? Apart from anything else, some of the rules governing patent medicine advertising are based on social convention, not on some grand moral or medical law; and in these circumstances it probably bespeaks a politically healthy society if some advertisers sail pretty close to the wind.

The types of contravention of the code can be grouped under certain headings, but they overlap one another a good deal; and the following five are certainly not exhaustive. They are listed here so that the reader may have a few concrete examples of advertising sin. And if the concrete should seem not to have set here and there, do please remember that I have to avoid naming or suggesting individual products: I shall do my best within those limits.

First, then, there is the kind of statement or implication that any doctor knows to be untrue, or largely untrue, but that is often very much in accord with popular belief. The most striking examples involve laxatives. Their advertisements suggest or state that we should use laxatives regularly for good health; that laxatives are needed to get rid of poisonous waste material from our bodies; and that, if we take laxatives, we shall have more of an appetite, more energy, and brighter eyes, and shan't get depressed. As we saw in Chapter 8, the great majority of doctors believe all this to be so much nonsense, as would anyone else who studied the matter. However, the general public has a different view – and the manufacturers side with the general public, their customers.

Second, there are statements or implications that have only a morsel of truth in them, though it is made to seem like a mountain. Thus there is no more than a grain of it in a statement that what is essentially a food will help one to get to sleep. Again, as far as doctors know, there is probably little truth in a suggestion that vitamins will protect people against colds; and the best available medical evidence suggests that only one kind of patent medicine aspirin causes less stomach bleeding than any other. Also, doctors are far from sure exactly what it is about aspirin that makes it produce indigestion in some people; but the advertisers of certain aspirin products can tell one – and do. And finally in this category; a tonic consisting largely of protein will *not* bring you back to health unless you're one of those very, very few people who cannot, for a time, face ordinary foods containing protein but can face a protein tonic.

Third, there are advertisements that imply superiority in a product when none at all exists. This may be by stating that it contains six (or ten or fifteen) separate ingredients: a doctor knows that any product containing more than a couple of active ingredients is usually suspect, but the man in the street does not know it. Again, despite what is said or implied in the advertisements, there is not a great deal of difference between the speeds of action of most patent medicine relievers, any differences are not very important in practice, and some of the big factors that could affect these speeds of action (for example, that, when the analgesic is taken, the stomach is full of food or empty) have nothing at all to do with the products themselves.

Fourth, there are advertisements that strongly imply that certain people *need* a particular kind of patent medicine product when they do not. The wording in these usually runs something like this: If you suffer from fatigue (depression, poor appetite, run-down feeling, etc., etc.), then you may be suffering from a lack of iron (vitamins, protein, minerals etc., etc.). Yes, you *may*. But what the advertisements omit to mention is that, although such symptoms *may* be due to a lack of vitamins or protein, they very rarely are, in fact, due to such a lack, at least in this country. They *are* due, much more often, to an iron lack; but, as we said in Chapter 14, people suffering from a lack of iron should be treated by their doctors, and not with iron-containing patent medicines.

And fifth, there are advertisements that mention pseudo-complaints or support their claims with pseudo-science. These, of course, are very common. The two most interesting pieces of pseudo-science I encountered during my scrutiny of advertisements were the implication that two hours after a meal the stomach should not contain any undigested food (in fact, if it doesn't, you probably *should* start worrying), and the statement that gases from a medicine can rise straight up from the stomach to the lungs: alas! those fuddy-duddy men, the doctors, who believe in observation and experiment, know that the contents of a medicine can go from stomach to lung in only one way – circuitously through the heart and blood stream. There is no short cut.

But now how is it that advertisements of these five kinds (and there are others) get published? In many cases it is the implication of the advertisement that contravenes the code, not any direct statement; and, of course, it is not difficult for the legalistic, hair-splitting type of mind to defend an alleged implication for a long, long time. And then it is nearly always possible to find *some* medical or scientific paper *some*where that will support almost any statement one cares to make. Indeed, doctors being highly individualistic, one can usually find a handful of doctors who hold views on a health topic that are diametrically opposed to those of 99·9 per cent of the profession. It is, of course, wrong to use such papers or such doctors to defend an advertisement, but it is done. And when the opinion of a tiny minority of doctors is the same as that of the great majority of lay people (as in the case of constipation and laxatives), it is particularly difficult to eliminate advertisements that make use of that opinion.

Nevertheless, in the case, for example, of laxatives, the Advertising Association's leaflet on their advertising (which is meant to supplement the *British Code*) states: 'There is little evidence to justify the traditional belief that a daily motion is essential or desirable for good health, or that ill effects necessarily result from longer intervals between evacuations. ... There is no evidence that the use of laxatives improves the complexion ... or produces bright eyes. ... There is no indication for the habitual use of laxatives without medical guidance.' How can one reconcile all this with what is being said or implied in some advertisements for patent medicine laxatives? I should be extremely interested to hear from anyone who is able to.

Of course, contraventions of the code are important, mainly, though not only, in so far as they promote unhealthy habits or instil ideas about health into people's minds that are not valid. What do patent medicine advertisements achieve in this respect? One can, of course, speak only in terms of probabilities; but what follows constitutes the most serious criticism that can be levelled against patent medicines, and provides doctors with their most valid reason for wanting to have nothing to do with them. Advertisements for patent medicines most probably do tend to make people think that the taking of medicines is necessary for a full and healthy life, and that the taking of medicines is harmless. They tend to make people take medicines for non-existent ailments, or for ailments that call for something other than medical treatment (perhaps a change of diet, or of work or else skilled psychiatric treatment), or for unnecessarily long periods, or for complaints, particularly chronic complaints, that should properly be treated by a doctor. Anyone who doubts that these effects occur should talk to some friends about patent medicines, and then compare what they believe with what can be learnt from this book about the truth as doctors see it.

Practically all of the ill effects mentioned are a natural consequence of much current advertising for laxatives, and various of them are a natural consequence of some current advertising for vitamin products, tonics, cough medicines, and analgesics. And most of them would be prevented if the present *British Code* were strictly applied in the case of every patent medicine advertisement. Here perhaps is the real hub of the case against the present arrangements for the control of patent medicine advertising: none of the bodies concerned with that control has real teeth that it regularly uses – and yet, to judge by their *own* standards, those that have teeth certainly should be using them.

It may be said that we don't want more control, that intelligent people will take all advertising with a big grain of salt, and indeed find patent medicine advertisements more of a joke than anything else. But unintelligent people have no monopoly of gullibility when it comes to matters of health: the cleverest and most distinguished can be taken in. A few years ago Queen Bee jelly enjoyed its best sales in shops catering for the most exclusive clientele in the country, and yet it is next door to useless. (I am not, of course, equating social exclusivity with intelligence, but there is perhaps some degree of correlation: one has to have a little native wit to grasp the idea of exclusivity.)

A more valid objection to any extension of existing controls on advertising is that it is demanded by various Do-Gooders, Busy-bodies, and other narrow-minded people who believe, to use a war-time phrase, that the gentlemen in Whitehall know best. They can see the mote in everyone's eye but their own, these people, especially in the eye of a businessman; they forgive nothing and they forget nothing; they see in exquisite detail to the ends of their noses – and no further! Indeed, in the last ten or fifteen years a minor profession has grown up, concerned with denigrating anything produced by industry, anything on which a profit is made, anything of which its sweating creator is proud and for which, being human, he beats a big drum.

Some of the criticisms of these people are nevertheless valid; and one cannot be deterred from recommending what is right by the fact that there are people supporting it for the wrong reasons. And I believe that a body should be set up by the Government, but independent of it, and independent too of manufacturers, media owners, advertising agents, Do-

Gooders, etc., that shall have the duty of continuously survey-
ing the field of patent medicine advertising and the power to
impose penalties for contraventions of an agreed advertising
code, which would probably be similar to the present *British
Code*. Such a body would probably have a part-time governing
body, and a full-time secretariat; the penalties it could impose
to be fairly severe, and to be quashable only by a High Court
judge. It would really be the advertising opposite number of
the Dunlop Committee, which deals with drug safety.

This body would not see *all* advertisements before they
were published: that would be quite impracticable, and unnecessary. Nor would it be required to scrutinize every single
published advertisement. It would 'vet' a substantial number of
published advertisements (keeping its method of selection of
them flexible and secret); and would have the power to
demand of any advertiser the proof for any statement he made,
or implication that was contained, in an advertisement; and
if it decided that the statement or implication constituted a
clear, and major, and intentional breach of the code, then a
severe penalty would automatically follow – say, for a statement
meant of set purpose to make people take a patent medicine in
such circumstances that the taking of it would quite probably
do harm, an interdict on any advertising of that product for a
period of twelve months. If a penalty of that severity were to
be imposed only two or three times a year, the standard of
patent medicine advertising would enormously improve in a
matter of months, and it would stay at its new-found level.

There would, of course, be difficulties in the way of prov-
ing intent, and in dealing with breaches of the spirit of the
code; but a little firm justice in the early days, and a good deal
of humanely administered justice subsequently – this would
soon remedy the worst of the present evils with a minimum of
hardship, or of damage to business enterprise.

Details aside, nobody who believes the present *British Code*
to be a reasonable one could object to such an arrangement;
and certainly, as far as manufacturers are concerned, the setting up of such a body would be preferable to what many of

the Do-Gooders in our midst would prefer – the complete abolition of the patent medicine industry. Having now looked at various means of improving it short of abolition, we are free in our next chapter to consider what might, in fact, be the result of making it vanish altogether.

*   *   *   *   *

The 1967 White Paper on drugs, mentioned in Chapter 19, which will doubtless lead to legislation taking effect in 1968, lays it down that advertisements for a drug that falsely describe it or might mislead are to be forbidden, and also advertisements containing claims going beyond those covered in the drug's licence. Steps will be taken to ensure that in a drug advertisement adequate information about the drug is provided. Doubtless much of the work in connection with this control of advertising will fall on the new Medicines Commission suggested in the White Paper. However, ultimate power, it seems, will reside with the Government, and this is one of the few features of this proposed new legislation that cannot be wholeheartedly welcomed.

22

Abolition or Reform?

THERE ARE quite a number of people who, without any hesitation, would say about patent medicines, 'Scrap the lot.' Some of them would be saying it because they have no time for any product of big business, particularly when a great deal of advertising is used to sell it; and others because some patent medicine advertisements are untrue or misleading, and militate against health. Others again have read and accepted all the criticisms that have been made over the years of the manufacturers of prescription-only drugs. They would be right to think that firms who are making 'ethical' medicines also make most of the patent medicines, and right to think that some part of the criticisms must have been justified. However, although we cannot go into any details here, the manufacturers of ethical drugs have sometimes, in fact, been made a whipping boy when the real fault lay elsewhere. And in any case, are the sins of a brother to be visited on his non-identical twin? Is the patent medicine industry to be liquidated because the ethical industry is alleged to have some major faults?

Another group of abolishers think we use too many drugs, and that what we need should be provided for us by our doctors, because they alone know all about the dangers of drugs. Another group is against the taking of 'artificial' chemicals in the form of drugs. Another group – but we could go on for ever, and all the time there is one very good reason why abolition of patent medicines is impracticable. To state and to accept it is not to deny the industry's excesses, or to deny that some changes should be made. It is, however, to take account of realities.

The reason is this. The favourite answer of the abolitionists to questions about the possible effects of abolition is that, after abolition, we should be getting all our drugs on a doctor's prescription. Now, if people *were* suddenly denied access to all home medicines, and a good number did go to their doctors instead (which probably would happen), the medical services of this country simply would not be able to deal with the greatly increased demands made upon them. Health Service chaos might result.

This is a danger that even some doctors appear not to be strikingly conscious of – although, as we have seen, many of them are critical of patent medicines, and some of them would like all drugs to be obtainable only on prescription. It is nevertheless a very real danger, particularly at the moment and for a few years ahead.

What could happen if people turned to their doctors every time they were ill was well illustrated a few years ago during a 'flu epidemic. One patent medicine manufacturer put out a special television commercial, which told people that, if they got 'flu, they should take a dose of his pain-reliever, then go to bed, and call their doctor. Having made it, the manufacturer sat back feeling rather pleased with himself. Had he not, after all, succeeded in combining a plug for his product with a plug for the doctors? Surely this time they'd be happy.

Hardly, however, had the commercial been shown for the first time than there was an outcry from the doctors. They were, they said, completely overwhelmed by calls from 'flu victims. People who normally would have treated themselves from start to finish of their illness had taken the manufacturer's message to heart, and after one dose of his medicine had called the doctor and retired to bed. Doctors were getting dozens of *extra* calls a day. Their protests were understandable, and so loud that the commercial was very quickly withdrawn.

Well now, *do* doctors want to treat *all* illnesses, or do they want people to treat minor ailments themselves with freely available patent medicines? And, 'flu epidemics aside, what, in fact, would happen if there were no patent medicines for people to take? Let us try and answer this very important question.

The current annual cost of National Health Service prescriptions in England and Wales is about £150 million. The amount spent on patent medicines has been estimated at £70 million. Almost certainly, however, that £70 million represents a great many more individual episodes of illness than the £150 million. This is because prescription-only drugs are, in general, a good deal more costly than patent medicines: the cost of an average N H S prescription is ten shillings, which is a lot more than the average person spends at the chemist's on a remedy for his cold or headache or indigestion.

In addition, a single purchase of a household remedy is often used to treat, not one episode of illness, but several. It can be used repeatedly because the label on the container says what is in it. Prescription medicines, however – unless they are being taken for a chronic condition – are rarely used on more than one occasion because not even a doctor can readily tell you what is in a container simply labelled 'The tablets' or 'The medicine'. As a result, a lot of prescribed medicines are thrown away after a first period of usage. (And, if patent medicines were abolished, this sort of labelling might obtain for the prescribed drugs, however simple, provided in replacement.) Also, prescription drugs are free: patent medicines cost the individual money, and so are used more economically. And lastly, patent medicines are much more often taken in isolated doses, or perhaps only for a single day, than are prescribed medicines.

It would probably be a conservative estimate to say, on this basis, that there are twice as many episodes of illness treated with patent medicines as are treated with prescription medicines. Now suppose that, because there were suddenly no patent medicines, just half of these episodes resulted in a visit to the doctor. That seems a reasonable estimate. What would be the effect? Ask any family doctor: If his present number of new patients expecting prescriptions was doubled, not just when there was a 'flu epidemic, but year in, year out, he would certainly be unable to deal with them. The National Health Service might well collapse.

An estimate can be made in other ways. It is known that at any one time about three people are taking a patent medicine for every one who is taking a medicine prescribed by a doctor. Suppose only half the patent medicine takers would go to their doctors if patent medicines were no longer available: the number of new patients wanting a doctor's prescription would still be a good deal more than doubled.

Another estimate has it that three out of every four people suffer from some ailment each month, and that at present three out of every four people who do suffer from an ailment do not go to their doctor about it. What action *do* they take? About half of the ailments apparently don't get any treatment at all, but the remainder are presumably treated with patent medicines, and perhaps half of these would result in a visit to the doctor if there were no patent medicines available. So, as you will agree if you think about these figures, it seems on this basis also that the number of new patients wanting prescriptions from their family doctors would be about doubled if patent medicines were abolished.

It is true there is a lot of supposition, and even opinion, involved in these estimates; but however one looks at the problem, the conclusion is much the same: if the patent medicine industry suddenly ceased to exist, doctors would probably be overburdened to the point of breakdown.

It may be objected that it wouldn't take the doctor very long to treat the simple little illnesses for which people give themselves aspirin and so on. It wouldn't *really* add much to the doctor's work. Alas! if only it were true that a doctor could, simply by glancing at his patients, divide them straight away into the more serious and the less serious. But he can't. It's not even as though all of the new patients would helpfully say: 'I've nothing serious the matter with me, Doctor. I've come to you because I can't buy anything at the chemist's any longer.' Their attitude would often be the same as that of most patients now: 'I'm ill, Doctor. Make me well.'

To a doctor a headache may be just a headache, but it *can*, he knows, be a sign of something very serious. A cough may just be the end result of a cold, or it may be the first sign of a grave chest disease. A doctor's conscience will not allow him to jump to immediate conclusions about a patient: he feels that he must ask some questions, must nearly always carry out *some* examination, must usually arrange to see the patient again. But even if he could bring himself to take just a very quick look at each of his hypothetical new influx of patients, and at once write out a prescription for aspirin or whatever he thought was suitable, he would still most probably be unable to cope with the extra work. And he certainly wouldn't sleep easy at night.

Somebody else is doubtless saying that it wouldn't happen all of a sudden, this disappearance of patent medicines: we'd have at the very least a few months' notice; we'd be able to make plans. Well, if what this optimistic person has in mind is plans involving the doctors, let us be quite clear that there just aren't enough for the health plans existing at present, let alone for any new ones; nor will there be enough in the fore-seeable future.

The general public in this country is largely unaware that we have a severe shortage of doctors at present, and that it may well get worse. The number of doctors actually in charge of general practices is going down. In the hospitals of Great Britain there are some 4,000 Commonwealth doctors, many of them from India or African countries. If for any reason they decided to leave this country (and there are signs that the supply is now drying up), the hospital service would un-doubtedly collapse. Of recent years 400 doctors trained in the medical schools of Great Britain and Ireland have been emi-grating *every year*. This is about one quarter of the total annual output of doctors from our medical schools. These are facts. The reasons behind them are not relevant here.

Training more doctors is no solution, at least in the near future, because it takes a minimum of seven years to train a doctor. Most doctors would say that ten years was nearer the mark. It has been estimated that the hospital service alone will call for an extra 5,000 doctors in the next few years, but there is no hope at all of its getting this number. There is little doubt, in fact, that, if it were decided to ban, or greatly cut down, the use of patent medicines in this country, visits to the doctor would not be a possible substitute.

Could pharmacists provide the answer? What we have really been considering so far is the abolition of *all* home medicines, not just patent medicines. Suppose the pharmacist was left free to sell us his 'chemist's own' and standard remedies: he would then obviously be called upon to give advice on his medicines, for there would be no advertisements for them and no easy-to-remember brand names. However, advice on drugs cannot be separated from advice on health, and British pharmacists are at present working out their attitude to the idea of their becoming health educators, as well as purveyors of drugs. Quite probably they will decide to take on this role, which certainly needs to be filled. However, any decision-taking will be gradual, and in any case it would be some years before the effects could become obvious in most pharmacies.

So much for the possibility of doctors or even pharmacists being able to provide any immediate substitute for patent medicines if the latter were suddenly abolished by law. Many readers, however, may have been thinking to themselves that, if abolition did occur, hole-in-the-corner manufacture of home medicines, and under-the-counter sales of them, would occur – as well, probably, as increased visits to the doctor. They are almost certainly right, for, as we shall see in our next chapter, home medication has deep and powerful roots, and a long history. Would the abolitionists really like to see completely uncontrolled manufacture and sale of drugs, rather than an attempt to remove abuses in the present arrangements? Can their imaginations not tell them what might happen?

Some readers may think all of this represents a counsel of despair: we must not abolish patent medicines for fear of producing something even worse. But this implies that abolition is desirable, whereas most people, having read the last few chapters, will probably agree that, while there *are* defects in patent medicines and while various reforms *are* desirable, there is no good case (practicability aside) for anything so drastic.

Let us, for the sake of any doubters, bring together the main revisionist features of the last few chapters. We thought that the Committee on Safety of Drugs, or its successor, should be enabled to take a retrospective look at all patent medicines, and that submission to it of proposed new remedies should be compulsory. We felt there should be – and there almost certainly will be – legislation designed to improve manufacturing conditions, and to ensure that all patent medicines were made to certain high standards. Only for firms carrying out research and/or development work on new products would there be a future in the patent medicine industry. Labelling of patent medicines should be in English. There should be an advertising control body, which would scrutinize published advertisements for patent medicines, and would have power to apply sanctions for any contravention of an agreed code.

Finally, and most important of all, we felt that doctors should, of set purpose, advise and guide the industry, and that they should increase the amount of personal health education they give the public – in particular, in this context, on those topics knowledge of which would lead to a more discriminating and sensible usage of patent medicines. Increased health education is one of the most important steps of all, and, as it will be involved in one further big item of reform, which will be mooted at the end of this chapter, let us have a quick look at the subject.

This book itself is a small essay in health education; and of course, the amount of readily available information on health matters has increased greatly in the last ten or fifteen years – chiefly because, as part of a general change in our society, taboos on the open discussion of a number of subjects have been discarded: we can now talk about sex, about religion, and about health and disease much more freely than twenty or thirty years ago. Another reason is that the popular press, the cinema, radio, and, most important of all, television, have given us new eyes and ears, and we have demanded that they be used freely. And then new techniques and new drugs, discovered in this century, have made cure or relief possible for many previously intractable illnesses; and so doctors, no longer needing mumbo-jumbo and a bedside manner to conceal their inability to help, have much more often felt able to be frank with their patients.

Certainly the public has an insatiable appetite for information on doctors, health, disease, and drugs. This is perhaps associated with the decline in religious belief: when you cease to believe in the next world, you become much more interested in how long you may expect to enjoy this one. Also, in this materialistic, self-seeking age, doctors are thought of, and respected, as being devoted to an ideal of service. They are looked upon as very powerful as well as dedicated; and like children in relation to their parents, lay people want to probe what they believe to be the secret of that power and that dedication.

Not all doctors agree with the trend towards increased knowledge on health matters, and on all things medical. However, a Joint Committee of the Central and Scottish Health Services Council (sometimes known as the Cohen Committee after its doctor chairman, and containing seven doctors among its twelve members) came out very strongly in favour of more health education in its 1964 report on this topic. They proposed the expenditure of an extra half a million pounds a year, and the setting up of a new profession of Health Educators and of a new Health Education Council which, in fact, did eventually begin to operate in April, 1968. Indeed, there is no doubt that health education is here to stay, and is going to increase, and that a majority of doctors are in favour of education of the right sort. Some of the extra money to be spent on it could well be used in educating people in the matter of patent medicines, even though continuing personal education by the family doctor remains the most important element in this respect.

In its report that very distinguished committee had itself

something to say about patent medicines: 'A particular obstacle to progress is the belief that medicines, either self-prescribed or prescribed by a doctor, are necessary to regain or preserve health. This belief, which is encouraged by the commercial advertising of proprietary preparations, obscures the very important contribution which people may make to promoting their own health. ... The public, through health education, must be helped to evaluate the claims made by advertisers.'

And now I wish to put forward a major proposal, affecting patent medicine advertising, that might be of very great importance for health education and so might provide a partial answer to the grave shortage of doctors. My proposal is that it should become the rule – perhaps even by law – for patent medicine manufacturers to devote some agreed, substantial proportion of the space in all advertisements and leaflets to a health education item, which would be liable to the same scrutiny and control as the advertisement itself. An advertisement for an analgesic, for instance, might contain information on the common cause of headaches, and how to avoid them; or else on the choice of an analgesic by someone suffering from indigestion. A leaflet on a deodorant might contain information on personal hygiene. An advertisement for an antacid could give details of a diet suitable for the person prone to indigestion. And so on. A little information of this kind is provided now by some patent medicine manufacturers, but there is room for a very greatly increased provision of it and for an improvement of its quality.

We have seen in this chapter that there is a grave doctor shortage, and as general practitioners are burdened, among much else, with a host of petty complaints (so that on occasion they have not enough time to deal properly with the serious ones), surely doctors should jump at the chance, first, of advising the patent medicine manufacturers (as was suggested in Chapter 18), and second, of having them use their advertising skill and space, as now proposed, in the cause of health education. Doctors would be both getting rid of what they dislike in patent medicines and their advertisements, *and* seeing their patients educated in the self-management of minor disorders – thus diminishing their own work load.

But would the manufacturers co-operate voluntarily in these two respects? Well, as one consequence of the arrangement, they would certainly have the medical profession as friends, or at least as well-disposed neutrals, instead of as enemies; and that would be a considerable gain. As another consequence, most of the criticisms levelled against the patent medicine industry would become invalid; and the industry would thus be assured of immunity from abolition, nationalization, and all the other bogies that now have the chairmen and managing directors sleeping uneasily at night. These would be major gains. And the diehards in the industry might reflect that they were simply having to go along with the great social trends of our time – more information for the man in the street, greater consumer protection, a greater sense of responsibility on the part of the bosses in our economy.

One or both parties may well reject this suggested double co-operation between industry and profession, which is this book's chief contribution to a solution of the problems facing the industry (and incidentally to certain problems facing the medical profession). It will, however, be a great pity if they do not at least consider the suggestions carefully and with goodwill. After all, there is a third and more important party that is interested and that will be watching, however patiently – the general public.

23

A Longer, Deeper Look

WHY, WHEN they are ill or feel that they might be ill, do people take *patent* medicines? One reason obviously is because they're convenient: you can buy them at the chemist's round the corner, you know just what they're for, and you can keep them handy round the house for when next you need them. If you have a minor complaint, it's easier to take a patent medicine than to go to the doctor. Sometimes also people take a patent medicine because they are afraid to go to a doctor or because they have been disappointed with the results of his treatment.

But might there not be some other reason, deeper than any of these? What do patent medicines really mean to people? After all, everyone knows that a great many wonderful new drugs have been discovered in the past twenty or thirty years, most of them prescription-only; and that doctors are well trained and knowledgeable. So why do most people who are taking a prescribed medicine (which is free) also take a patent medicine (which costs money)? Why not be satisfied with what the doctor prescribes for us? The answer to these questions will take us right down to fundamentals.

Until the last 150 or 200 years most of the people of this country lived on or near the land. If they were ill, especially if they had minor illnesses, they relied on homely remedies, particularly herbal remedies, the ingredients and virtues of which were known through the lore of folk medicine – a collection of myths, half-baked science, and other irrationalities. However, people did feel at home with those remedies. They might be mysterious in their action, but they were familiar; and because they were mysterious they might also be magical. And in a way they were human as well – in scale and in character. Much the same could be said about the illnesses themselves, as well as about the remedies: mystery and magic figured in *them* also, and many of them were thought to have a quasi-human quality, which made them familiar, if terrible. It is not very long since people were 'possessed by devils'; and since nobody thought it odd to see a picture portraying the Captains of the Men of Death.

The view that people two centuries ago had of life in general was similar to the view they had of illness. Living close to the land, they were all the time surrounded by its beauty and mystery and magic, as well as by its cruelty and ugliness. However, for all its virtues and its faults, it was on much the same scale as man, and it operated in the same way as man himself operated, or as he thought he did. It was warm and alive. Even the mysteries were governed by forces, often personalized, that would respond to the same kind of influence as swayed man himself. Even to God, Who had created and governed it all, you talked as you would to another man. Man, in one form or another, was at the centre of it all.

And then Manchester and Salford were built, and Leeds and Sheffield, and Bolton and Blackburn and Bradford. Wherever the people looked there were dirty bricks and stones instead of grass or mud. Instead of John Barleycorn, or Jack Frost, there was a big cotton mill, full of efficient but inhuman machinery. One could see exactly how it worked, even though one didn't understand every detail. There was no mystery, and certainly no magic: it would turn out just so many thousands of items a day, no more, no less. And there was no real change as the nineteenth-century city of grimy brick became the twentieth-century city of glass and concrete.

In either century this new world was a hard, cold, inhuman one, for all its efficiency. Nobody liked it greatly. However, everyone could understand it: everyone could read (after a time), and there were schools in the cities, and libraries, and newspapers, and in the end films and broadcasting. And from them people learned about machines and about science. And those who learned very little? Well, they at least accepted that it was quite possible to learn a lot more.

And so in time the people came to realize that the world is not of human scale, and does not work in the same way as man's mind works. The world, they found, is a speck in the universe, which is not even hostile to man. If it were, one might feel happier: an enemy can become a friend, but something that is coldly non-human can never be anything else. And the universe apparently was cold and non-human, governed by the simple, logical laws of science.

Strangest of all, man himself was governed by them. You felt ill for straightforward reasons – cold, hard, and straightforward reasons. Anyone who received the right training could understand them. Also, such a person could tell you how long you probably had to live – on average, of course, not as an individual. And the treatment for illness was equally cold and hard and logical. A chemical in a test tube. A little white tablet. An X-ray or some other kind of ray coming out of a machine. An operation that was simply like a very delicate bit of plumbing. They'd even operate on your brain at times, and then you might find you were a different person. They could do all kinds of things, wonderful things really; but there were quite definitely no miracles any longer, and no mysteries that science couldn't one day solve. And naturally there was no God to talk to. Not any longer. He was not needed.

That description of what has happened to man as a result of our industrial and scientific revolution is very short, and there are doubtless some half-truths in it, and some omissions, and many simplifications. Nevertheless the broad picture it presents is valid. And there is no doubt that man, or a part of him, has not liked the substitution of a laboratory for the magic wand of his fairy tales, or a real jet plane for the magic carpet of his dreams. He has not liked his new, cold, logical, scientific world, even though he has himself striven to create it. It is one thing to have a vision, another to see it realized.

The dislike is not often admitted openly. After all, most of the material side of our lives was created by modern scientific method, and depends on scientific method for its everyday running. However, one sign of the dislike is the undoubted existence of two cultures in our society. It is no disgrace – indeed, it is one element in a truly aristocratic *hauteur* – to claim to be completely ignorant of science, whereas most 'educated' people would be ashamed to admit they knew nothing at all about Shakespeare or about history.

I am not defending this antagonism towards science (which extends to science's twin, industry, as well), nor am I attacking it. I am merely stating that it exists. How long it will continue to exist is a matter of opinion. Some people think that, with increasing scientific education in our schools and universities, it will have vanished in a couple of generations. More probably, I suggest, it is a product of a very powerful irrational element in human nature, and will not be eradicated at all quickly – unless, of course, science itself discovers a means of eradicating it. In fact, science probably will discover a means, perhaps an unpleasant one. And my own latent bias against science is shown by my use of the word 'unpleasant'. Why should I not have assumed that the means might be pleasant, or at least neutral?

Man's bias is understandable, of course. After all, until yesterday he was living in essentially the same way and with the same mental approach to life as had served humanity for thousands of generations: and it really would be too much to expect that he should suddenly discard these completely, or that they would not in many ways correspond to something strong and important in his make-up. His body, as we can see from the new diseases afflicting it, was not made for the motor car, and for the refrigerator constantly full of food; and his mind is no different.

But now what exactly has this to do with patent medicines? I suggest that patent medicines have been one of the means – inadequate though they are, and even pathetic – that the man in the street has used as links with his old life, and as outlets for the emotions and ways of thought associated with that life. In a small way they have helped to supply a mystery and magic, a hope, a sense of life and of power that were absent from the black industrial cities of the nineteenth century, and are just as much absent from the bright scientific ones of the twentieth. Patent medicines have provided a small refuge in the cold world that science has created; with their help, even though there were no gardens, the nineteenth-century man in the street could at least – even in the back alleys of Manchester and Leeds – always cultivate himself. It is not so fantastic: 'As others gardens, they themselves do tend', one poet wrote.

Patent medicines, after all, reached their peak of popularity, if not sales, at the end of the last century. It was then, too, that advertising of them showed its wildest excesses. And they were most popular of all in the densely populated industrial regions of the North – in Lancashire and Yorkshire. Even today there are probably more old-established patent medicine manufacturers to be found in the towns of Yorkshire and Lancashire than anywhere else in the country. At the same time one of the most popular claims for a patent medicine has always been that it was 'natural' or 'Nature's Own' – harking back, surely, to the era of herbals.

And certainly patent medicines have always been mysterious: even today the ingredient names on the packet are in very small type, and not one person in a hundred knows what the names mean – though many people read them, as they might read an incantation in a strange language. And patent medicines do have magic properties. Until recently their manufacturers were saying so themselves, quite openly: patent medicines dissolved away whatever it was had caused the pain, they would attack and destroy the excess of acid or the lurking germs or the first hard deposits of old age. You could read all about it: you had been taught to read – if only a newspaper.

Patent medicines are still magical today – if more quietly proclaimed to be so – whereas the doctor's medicines are limited in their effects, however powerful those effects may be. And it is relevant that even doctors, or many of them, when they are at all seriously ill, like to lie back in bed and be told by a colleague just what to do and what not to do. They like to be given some tablets and to be instructed to take one every four hours and two at bedtime. And they don't really like to be told what is in the tablets. They like their touch of magic too.

Indeed, perhaps the basic distinguishing feature of patent medicines has always been that they hold out the promise of enabling one to live for ever: scientific medicine merely tells one just how many years one can expect on average, and how to be, with luck, a little above the average. Who, deep down, wants that sort of medicine? Who wants to understand just why in the end there is no cure, rather than believing that there always must be a cure? Who doesn't want a magic medicine? Alas! very few of us. Truth is too strong a draught when death is the flavouring of it.

One or two objections to this thesis can be put forward. For instance, it could be said that the reason for the great popularity of patent medicines in the last century was simply the combination of misery and semi-literacy in the industrial cities: people were ignorant and took patent medicines, like alcohol, almost as a means of escape, believing all that their advertisements said about them. Even though this is true, is it not just another way of saying that patent medicines, if they didn't represent any harking back, were certainly regarded as magical and hopeful? And it cannot have been the major reason for their popularity, even in the nineteenth century, because that popularity has continued into the seventh decade of *this* century, and our society is affluent and fairly sophisticated (even though it may have its own brand of misery beneath the surface). Sales of patent medicines go up almost every year, and this at a time when it is possible to obtain any needed medicines free under the National Health Service.

A second possible objection is that the drug revolution has occurred only in the last thirty to forty years. How could people in the last century have had any distaste for a 'scientific' medicine that didn't then exist? Well, although it is true that the great changes in drug treatment have come about only in the last few decades, the nineteenth century saw the introduction of anaesthetics, of the germ theory of disease, and of many complex surgical techniques, not to speak of various major discoveries in science and technology with which medicine was quite rightly associated in people's minds. The nineteenth century saw medicine become scientific; and above all, it was pregnant with most of the discoveries of the twentieth century and knew it was. Men sensed that a great change had come. Certainly, drug treatment aside, the nineteenth-century doctor was almost as scientific in his approach as his twentieth-century successor, and his philosophy was completely different from that of the vendors of patent medicines.

A third objection is that nineteenth- and twentieth-century man has favoured 'chemical' pills and potions, rather than the herbal remedies that my thesis would lead one to expect. But apart from the fact that herbal elements, albeit in token quantities, are still found in some 'chemical' patent medicines, this was surely because the 'chemical' remedies were easy to manufacture in bulk – by making use of the new scientific manufacturing techniques. (One cannot produce 100 tons of a herb to order, or treat it as one may a chemical.) Science, in other words, both created a problem and suggested the mechanics of a partial solution to it.

It is an irony of the situation altogether, indeed, that most of today's patent medicines are minor products of the very industrial, scientific, and medical revolution against which I believe them to be widely, if secretly, regarded as a defence; and that the advertising for them has borrowed the phraseology, and the graphs and the diagrams of science. But then they are not really graphs and diagrams at all, and the phrases do not mean what the scientists mean by them: science in the patent medicine advertisements is transformed into a thing of mystery and magic. The advertisements have simply replaced the old-time stories of fairies and hobgoblins; and their science is simpler and more human than science proper ever can be. At the same time the strength of science – which, after all, no one can deny – is made familiar and obedient, instead of being remote and dominating. Science has become the biggest magic ingredient in the majority of patent medicines.

The manufacturers and their advertising agents, down-to-earth and even cynical though some of them may be, do not give their products this kind of image in *full* awareness of what they are doing. Tell a modern advertising man that he is a teller of up-to-date fairy tales, and he may give you a rude answer. But this does not at all alter the truth of the position. Many manufacturers and advertising men are themselves very credulous in private – even over products they are very familiar with, and about which they have been cynical five minutes before in the committee room. It is faith, present both in these men and in the general public, that sustains much of the patent medicine industry. Faith, after all, is an even better healer than time; and man always yearns for something or someone he can have complete faith in. For one segment of his life – a smallish segment perhaps – patent medicines fill the bill.

If what has been said is substantially true, what conclusions should one draw? If you're an extremely rational person, especially if you're a scientifically minded one, you may draw the conclusion that, if patent medicines really are taken to any extent for the kind of reasons suggested, then the sooner they're abolished the better. But one should surely be careful about getting rid of something, however small its intrinsic value, that is playing a major part in people's lives – so long, at any rate, as it is not doing much harm. One never knows what the result may not be. And it has certainly not been established that patent medicines do a *great* deal of harm, and they obviously do some good. Perhaps, therefore, any reforming zeal one may have might be better turned to improving their usage than to abolishing them. This is, of course, to leave on one side the question, considered in the last chapter, of whether, in view of the doctor shortage, abolition is even a practical proposition.

There are, I suggest, two other and more important conclusions to be drawn from this amateur essay into mass motivation. First, if the desire for patent medicines *is* very deep-rooted, then health education will probably not produce any dramatically

quick changes in the public's attitude to them; and any reforms that will radically alter the 'image' of patent medicines should, of set purpose, be introduced gradually – many
of them (including most of those put forward in this book)
are, after all, the reforms of rational, science-minded,
twentieth-century man, and so could destroy something of what
the man in the street finds most attractive in his patent medicines.

Second, to be fully effective, health education may have to
adopt techniques similar to those used in the promotion of such
medicines. It may have to develop a 'magic' of its own. Much
health education is staid and unemotional – and so makes little
impact. Its protagonists have taken the word 'education' too
much to heart. 'Health motivation' or 'health propaganda'
would be better terms for what has to be done. And whatever
views one may have of the proper social scope of advertising,
there is no doubt that advertising men know best how to influence most people for the least cost in the shortest time. They
are the experts. The fact that one finds some advertisements
brash or garish or intolerably coy is as irrelevant as it would
be to object to a surgeon because, in one's ignorance, one did
not like the look of the instruments he was proposing to use on
one.

*　　　*　　　*　　　*　　　*

Those deep and speculative notes having been sounded, we
have almost reached the last page. And some readers may object that, despite any changes that may be produced by legislation, this book seems all the time to be envisaging, as a central
feature of the patent medicine scene, a continuing state of
tension between the manufacturers and their supporters on the
one hand and the critics of patent medicines on the other.
This is true, even allowing for some new legislation and a considerable degree of co-operation between the industry and the
medical profession; but such a state of tension is probably
healthy when any controversial issue is in question.

It is tempting to think there is a right way to do everything, and only one right way; and that people should be given no opportunity to choose any way but that. However, apart from considerations of people's right to freedom of choice or of the possibility that the initial choice of the 'right way' may be a mistaken one, it does seem that, once any individual or small group of individuals is given the power to choose a course for others to follow, and the power to keep them on that course, abuse nearly always results. That is why in any one field, when all generally accepted major abuses have been eliminated, and the various parties have been given the chance of fairly matched combat, it is best to let them play out the game with one another. It is not an easy way for the zealot to accept, but it seems to work very well in practice.

At the moment those who are critical of the patent medicine industry can probably make out a better rational case than its defenders. But what would happen if one gave them their head? Would it not be preferable gradually to strengthen their arm in the various ways that have been suggested or implied already, and then leave them and their opponents to hammer out a *modus vivendi* – which will change from year to year, from decade to decade, until at last the whole argument becomes meaningless and is replaced by another that we cannot now imagine?

That is surely the right way to deal with the situation – at least if one has respect for man, but does not always trust individual men. This book could clearly be a weapon in the hands of the reformers, but it was not meant to be, nor does it pretend to be the only repository of wisdom on the topic of patent medicines. It is a contribution to a continuing argument; and if it has brought some enlightenment to the average reader, and perhaps here and there a little hope to him, and a little strengthening of resolve, it will have served its purpose.

Index to Ingredients

A SELECTION OF POPULAR READING IN PAN

- [ ] **PRIDE AND PREJUDICE** Jane Austen   3/6
- [ ] **INHERITANCE** Phyllis Bentley   7/6
- [ ] **SHOOTING SCRIPT** Gavin Lyall   5/-
- [ ] **WUTHERING HEIGHTS** Emily Brontë   3/6
- [ ] **THE SOUND OF THUNDER** Wilbur A. Smith   6/-
- [ ] **ONE OF OUR SUBMARINES** Edward Young (illus.)   5/-
- [ ] **ROSEMARY'S BABY** Ira Levin   5/-
- [ ] **EAGLE DAY** Richard Collier (illus.)   6/-
- [ ] **THE MAN WITH THE GOLDEN GUN** Ian Fleming   3/6
- [ ] **THE SPY WHO LOVED ME** Ian Fleming   3/6
- [ ] **THE MAGUS** John Fowles   8/6
- [ ] **FRUIT OF THE POPPY** Robert Wilder   5/-

- [ ] **I CAN SEE YOU BUT YOU CAN'T SEE ME**
  Eugene George   5/-
- [ ] **THE ROOM UPSTAIRS** Monica Dickens   5/-
- [ ] **A SENTENCE OF LIFE** Julian Gloag   6/-
- [ ] **ON FORSYTE 'CHANGE** John Galsworthy   5/-
- [ ] **FAR FROM THE MADDING CROWD**
  Thomas Hardy   5/-
- [ ] **THE RELUCTANT WIDOW** Georgette Heyer   5/-
- [ ] **FREDERICA** Georgette Heyer   5/-
- [ ] **STRANGERS ON A TRAIN** Patricia Highsmith   5/-
- [ ] **STORIES MY MOTHER NEVER TOLD ME (Part I)**
  Alfred Hitchcock   3/6
- [ ] **YOUNG BESS** Margaret Irwin   5/-
- [ ] **THE DEEP BLUE GOOD-BYE** John D. MacDonald   3/6
- [ ] **THE LIFE OF IAN FLEMING**
  John Pearson (illus.)   7/6
- [ ] **SHAMELADY** James Mayo   3/6
- [ ] **MADONNA OF THE SEVEN HILLS** Jean Plaidy   5/-
- [ ] **ROUND THE BEND** Nevil Shute   5/
- [ ] **THE BOSTON STRANGLER** Gerold Frank   7/6

Obtainable from all booksellers and newsagents. If you have any difficulty, please send purchase price plus 6d. postage to PO Box 11, Falmouth, Cornwall.

I enclose a cheque/postal order for selected titles ticked above plus 6d. per book to cover packing and postage.

NAME _____

ADDRESS _____

_____